MORE MAGIC OF THE MINIMUM DOSE

MORE MAGIC OF THE MINIMUM DOSE

EXPERIENCES AND CASES

by
Dr DOROTHY SHEPHERD

The C. W. Daniel Company Limited
1 Church Path,
Saffron Walden, Essex

This Edition, completely revised and reset,
February 1974
Reprinted 1980
Reprinted (in paperback) 1995

ISBN 0 85207 299 6

Printed in Great Britain by
HILLMAN PRINTERS
(Frome) Ltd.

CONTENTS

FOREWORD TO THIRD EDITION

In revising Dr. Dorothy Shepherd's book, I have been constantly reminded of her complete dedication to the art and science of Homoeopathy which she knew to be a medicine of greater curative value than that of the allopathic school in which she was originally trained.

Her practice was a large one, and she drew patients to her from all walks of life, thus her experience in the cure of disease whether acute or chronic covered a wide field. Some of the chapters in this book are her personal experience, and all others are actual cases treated homoeopathically by Dr. Shepherd herself, either privately or in one of the clinics she regularly attended.

Few homoeopathic doctors make time to record the history of the varied cases of disease they deal with, thereby denying the lay public knowledge of the principles and practices of this art of medical treatment. Indeed many people even today are unaware that these safer ways to deal with the sickness and frailty of the human being are existent.

In a world that appears to be increasingly materialistic, the symptoms of ill health are correspondingly complex. The need for medicines that will deal with the mental and emotional states of life and safely restore the disturbed balances, recreating a sense of harmony and well being, becomes more and more an urgent necessity. Homoeopathy can and does fill this need.

Dorothy Shepherd always felt that much of the future of Homoeopathy lay in the hands of the ordinary man-in-the-street. By his demand for safer alternative medication in his time of need, when hope was well nigh lost, the homoeopathic art would be kept alive by those doctors and intelligent lay practitioners who truly sought to heal the sick. This book, once more brought before the intelligent reader, will, I hope, do much towards this end. If only more perceptive doctors are drawn to make a study of this great science, Dr. Shepherd's life and work will not have been in vain.

Her knowledge and wisdom of all aspects of life has

been generously shared through her writings over the years, and those readers who have collected her published works will rejoice to know that there are still fragments being gathered together for future publication which will bring further knowledge to those who faithfully follow the homoeopathic path.

GWENETH E. ROBINSON
Thornbury, N. Devon

CHAPTER ONE

SOME INTRODUCTORY REMARKS

The title *More Magic of the Minimum Dose* was chosen with deliberate intent, not only to allure and attract in this age of advertisement, but to open the door to the inner meaning of the mysteries of the art of true healing. Not magic as standing for wizardry or witchcraft, to which this ancient word has degenerated in our times, but as expounding the higher wisdom of the Magis or Masters of the mystery schools; wisdom as opposed to knowledge, which means something learned, a concrete fact: wisdom is higher knowledge, a step higher and further upward towards the abstract and inner knowledge, the esoteric meaning of knowledge, if you like.

Orthodox medicine is based on the study and application of a collection of so-called facts obtained by the irrational method of mass experiments, which are constantly being altered and added unto. There is no continuity, no fixed law, no appeal to pure reason, the structure of the edifice of scientific medicine is based on the quicksands of experimentation on animals, and results obtained from test tubes in laboratories far removed from the actual contact with the complicated functions of the human body. Just to quote an example of this, Penicillin in the laboratories of the present masters of medicine, kills and destroys certain types of virulent micro-organisms grown in the test-tubes, hence, so the scientific mind argues, it is bound to destroy these virulent organisms in the human body, and cure the diseases caused by their toxins. What happens in actual fact? The living body and certain unknown biological factors in the body, assert themselves and in time a resistance to Penicillin may develop, and though this wonder drug, in theory, should kill the bacteria found in the body, as it conclusively kills them in the test tubes, it is not always so in practice.

Pencillin does wonders in many instances I know, but what about the Penicillin resistant cases, they are getting more common. But this does not deter our Scientists. They go round and round in circles, looking for the cure with their eyes glued to the microscopes hoping to find it in the test tubes, and neglecting to apply logic and pure reason to their experiments. They never see how worldly-minded their theories are. Their arguments are wrong to start with. So many premises are made, and high hopes are held out, only to be dashed to the ground repeatedly. A premise in Logic means: a proposition previously stated or proved for after-reasoning. The public is fooled, and the Doctors, blinded by the blinkers of scientific proofs, cannot and will not see the truth, that they have failed and will continue to fail in their object of curing disease, until they go back to the bed-side and learn by observation from the patient direct, what is wrong physiologically and how to cure it.

On the other hand Homoeopathy is purely a bed-side medicine and is based on a firm rock, the unalterable laws of healing, firstly the Law of Similarity, that Like cures Like — and secondly the Law of Potentisation, which means the law of producing power in the drug and thus energizing it. In other words the power of the minimum dose in arresting and curing disease which was proved biologically on the living organisms of healthy volunteers. The energies found in the emanations from radio-active substances have been recognized and have been applied in many different ways: physically and materially speaking such radio-active substances are quantitatively insignificant, but qualitatively their power is immense, in spite of their minuteness.

There are other subsidiary laws which explain and confirm the truth of homoeopathy and why it is vital and necessary for maintaining and upholding the health of mankind.

I do not deny that orthodox medicine does cure in some cases, it does relieve and palliate many conditions, the orthodox Doctor in rare cases experiences the great satisfaction of pulling a patient out of the jaws of death. The sulphonamides are the nearest approach to miracle workers, but they are so often applied indiscriminately, there is no law for their application, so frequently they do more harm than good and the bacteria appear to be getting wise and are developing sulphonamide resistant strains.

Not so long ago I had lengthy discussions with an orthodox Doctor of Medicine on Homoeopathy, and its results. He demanded proofs and comparative experiments, and denied that orthodox medical authorities were not just as keen as homoeopaths in curing people, or that they were unwilling to give homoeopaths the facilities of proving the truth of their statements. He was told that he should study the cases in homoeopathic hospitals, and that if homoeo-pathic doctors were given equal chances with other doctors as regards beds in general hospitals all over the country, soon the superiority of their methods would have to be acknowledged.

I could only show him one case on the spur of the moment, the rapidity with which Arnica taken internally in an infinitesimal dose had cured a large bruise on the forehead within a few minutes. All pain and swelling had disappeared in less than 20 minutes. All the answer I got was 'Did you have a control case'. But he did not respond when he was asked to be the control.

It is a pity that Logic is no longer a compulsory subject for medical men, for these worldly-minded scientists have long ago forgotten how to argue, if they ever knew. They are full of fixed ideas and they have forgotten the old saying 'Il n'y a pas des maladies seulement des malades' that is 'there is no sickness, only sick people, no diseases, only diseased people'. Homoeopathy does not cure diseases, only diseased people. There is no cure for Pneumonia, Influenza or Malaria as such; only a cure for individual people, suffering from Pneumonia maybe or Influenza or Malaria or any other disease. Mass experiments based on Homoeopathic principles are difficult to carry out, if you have no beds under your control — and when medical men as a body, are against anything which is not recognized by the governing majority. And yet, in acute cases Homoeopathy has a much greater recovery rate, and a much lower death roll, and its advantages could therefore be easily proved.

Speaking for myself, without any desire to blow my own trumpet — I am just stating facts — thanks to Homoeopathy and since I took it up and applied it I have never lost any cases suffering from Measles, Whooping Cough or Influenza, and none were ever sent to Hospital because they were too far gone. One case of alcoholic Broncho-Pneumonia in an elderly man died, and no other Pneumonia case was lost. All the acute infectious cases treated homoeopathically were cured rapidly, without any complications following. Many chronic, supposedly incurable cases were cured satisfactorily. There was a young lad who had suffered for years from bronchiectasis. Within a year of starting the treatment the large cavity in his lungs had completely closed up. He went back to the Radiologist who had previously X-rayed him, and when he saw on the plate that the cavity had disappeared, and that the lung was sound, he was delighted and interested, as he had never seen such a case before in his experience. When he was told this followed on Homoeopathic treatment, his interest waned completely.

A case of Ménières disease, progressive deafness with recurring attacks of giddiness and collapse was cured within a few weeks, the hearing became almost normal, with no return of giddiness and sudden collapses. Yet he had been told that nothing further could be done for him, and that his working days were over. True, he had only been ill for just over twelve months; it was not an advanced case, but the fact remains, Homoeopathy cured, where orthodox medicine could not, and held out no hopes for him either.

A case of high blood pressure in a middle-aged woman who had to have monthly blood lettings, so as to prevent the pressure from rising too high, and in spite of this was almost a complete invalid, who could not turn in bed without the greatest discomfort, and could not walk downstairs or stoop, for fear of these ghastly giddy turns, which threatened to engulf her, recovered quickly after having received Homoeopathic treatment, and three and a half years later she is so well that she can do a full day's work, dig the garden, stoop to her heart's content, and has never been back to the Hospital for any further blood-lettings, and the blood pressure has remained normal.

A girl of 26 who had been attending hospital for 15 years for steadily increasing obesity due to glandular deficiency, without receiving any benefit, after 9 months of Homoeo-pathic treatment lost 2½ stones in weight from 15 stones − 12½ stones, and has also lost her migraines, her aches and pains all over the body, her constipation is a thing of the past, and she is full of energy, feels well and looks well, and without any alteration in her diet and without Thyroid.

A case of generalized Xanthoma, an extremely rare case of multiple tumour formations underneath the skin, resembling pieces of yellow cartilage − who had been a show case at examinations for nearly twenty years, and where the tumours had been slowly spreading all over the body, under Homoeo-pathic treatment these nodules receded and are being dissolved. So that instead of having yellow tumours on his ear-lobes, his knees, his legs, his buttocks and arms, his skin is clearing beautifully, practically all have gone except for a few small lumps near his right elbow where the disease started first, and these nodules are getting steadily smaller and softer every month. These chronic cases require treatment for months and months, sometimes for years; these deep-seated complaints need careful treatment and prolonged supervision, but is it not worth-while?

A case of rheumatoid arthritis with so-called Heberden's nodules over the joints at the base of his fingers, which means according to prolonged observations that such a case is an incurable one, has so far cleared up in a year that these nodules have practically disappeared, the pain has gone, and the swellings and stiffness of the hands are greatly improved. He can now use his hands, he can mow his lawn which he has not been able to do for years, he is able to run up and down stairs, where previously he had to crawl up slowly and cautiously. He has given up the Aspirin long ago, which, though it had helped his pains and made life bearable, had not prevented the disease from spreading.

One cannot say that similar cases in other people will be cured by the same drugs which cured these cases I have just mentioned. Homoeopathy is a medicine for the individual, and the medicines given vary not with the name of the disease, but with the person suffering from the disease. Hence it is difficult to practise Homoeopathy, for it is an individualised medicine, not mass-controlled medicine. Whether Homoeopathy will survive, I do not know; it is not materialistic enough in this materialistic world of today, where men worship the State with a capital S instead of worshipping God; where spiritual truths are forgotten. The laws in the Kingdom of God are, 'Love thy God first', and then further, 'Love thy neighbour as thyself'. Not until man returns to God and to the divine spirit within himself, will he be free from the bondage of this material world and be able to make the fullest use of the Spiritualized medicine, which has been called Homoeopathy, the medicine based on the true Laws of Healing which few people, including doctors, understand or even try to understand.

CHAPTER TWO

THE BENEFITS OF HOMOEOPATHY

Homoeopathy is a wonderful thing and but rarely leaves you in the lurch, even though you are far removed from all the amenities of civilization, including hospitals and doctors. A personal experience may help to illustrate the advantage of Homoeopathy over other kinds of medical treatment, which generally presupposes a large surgical staff, antiseptics, sterilizing apparatus, hypodermics, antibiotics etc. One summer holiday, after a gorgeous day in the clear air of a Swiss mountain resort, I was wakened in the middle of the night by agonizing pains in the right foot, and in consequence passed a very restless and uncomfortable night. The next morning, on examining the foot, acute sepsis of one of the toes was found, which had spread up the foot, almost as far as the ankle, oedema, acute inflammation with a line of demarcation, the lymphatics were tender and outlined higher up. This meant a rapidly spreading sepsis and no surgical means at hand to combat it — nothing at all except a case of homoeopathic drugs. The foot was swollen and tender, it would not bear the pressure of a boot, even if there had been one large enough to fit over the dressing. The foot could not be put to the ground even. A nice predicament to be in! Miles away from the nearest postal coaching station — about two hours' walk over rough mountain paths and then sixteen miles by coach and three hours' journey by train to the nearest surgeon and hospital. Septicaemia sprang to mind. I remembered seeing cases dying within two or three days of neglected sepsis of the foot.

It was also remembered, however, that homoeopathic lotions were made from herbs of the fields and woods, and that the Almighty had given us all these things for our use, if we only cared to apply them. As I was unable to walk, a kind friend went out to collect some mountain Hypericum, or St. John's Wort. True, it was not the kind commonly used in Homoeopathy, which is the *H. perforatum*, but one had read that the leaves of another variety called *Tutsanor (toute saine) or H. androsaemum* were applied by the wise women in olden times to fresh wounds and to ulcerating and sloughing sores. With nothing else at hand, it was well worth trying. A bundle of the whole plants including the roots was collected and an infusion made by steeping it for a short time in boiling water. This produced an aromatic greenish liquor and a handkerchief was soaked in this hot lotion, wrung out and applied to the swollen foot. Relief quickly followed, whenever the dressing got dry it was damped afresh, usually at three hourly or four hourly intervals. By the evening distinct progress was noticed, the swelling was much less, the heat and pains were nearly gone, and by next morning, within twenty-four hours of starting treatment, it was possible to put the foot to the ground and limp downstairs. I continued the dressings for several days, and five days later the foot was well enough to go for walks again.

The external application of *Hypericum* was aided by internal medications of *Hep. Sulph. m*, alternately with *Hypericum m. Hep. sulph.* was given because of the great tenderness and the aversion to touch. It is very useful in early septic conditions and prevents abscess formation, and *Hypericum* was chosen as the condition started near the nail and might have been due to pressure of the heavy nailed mountain footgear. Thanks to homoeopathic knowledge and the use of a simple herb, I was saved a great deal of pain, a great deal of anxiety and incidentally expense. I shudder to think of the long, painful journey with a septic foot which might have had to be endured if it had not been for Homoeopathy. And yet doctors prefer the knife, prefer vaccines which are uncertain in their action, are really filthy and disgusting, if you only stop to think how they are made: by injecting a broth of pus germs into an animal, a horse usually, and then using some of the serum which is said to contain the protective immune substances to counteract the sepsis. A roundabout painful process, to both the horse and to yourself, as the resulting serum has to be drawn from the horse or rabbit or guinea pig and is then injected into the bloodstream, or into the tissues underneath the skin in order to do any good, which is problematical. I would rather make my own simple herbal lotions and use our homoeopathic remedies which are exact and are known to act as has been proved by years and years of clinical experience.

I never travel without a precious case of high dilution remedies and a god-send they have proved to me many times. In August, 1938, there was nearly a minor catastrophe: while travelling across France to Switzerland, a travelling companion was taken ill with sudden migraine, severe headache, fainting attacks, vomiting and collapse; and unfortunately the medicine case was packed away in the registered luggage. The train was hours late and the poor patient had to be taken in a collapsed condition up a mountain railway. At last after twelve hours of misery, I was able to get hold of the magic case; fortunately the luggage was not lost in transit! – and after a minute dose of *Ipecacuanha, m.* the patient revived, sat up, demanded and enjoyed a basin of hot soup and went sound asleep. In her pre-homoeopathic days this patient had suffered from these attacks for forty-eight hours at a time; now see how quickly one dose of *Ipecac.*, the indicated remedy, in the minutest quantity – acted. Next morning the dose of *Ipecac.* was repeated and the case cleared.

On another occasion, again in Switzerland, a friend was suddenly attacked with a variety of gastric influenza which was raging in that valley and in the Hotel, as we heard later. There was simultaneous sickness and diarrhoea, worse at night, worse between 1 and 2 a.m.; great restlessness and prostration and thirst. *Arsenic* seemed indicated and was given half-hourly because of the acuteness of the condition. However, *Arsenic* did not go deep enough, and it was found after watching the patient carefully that various other symptoms developed. In acute diseases symptoms change rapidly sometimes, as the disease develops. The *Arsenic* stopped the vomiting and the nausea, but did nothing for the inflammation of the bowels. The diarrhoea continued: the stools were dark brown, thin and fluid, occasionally mixed with a little blood, extremely foetid and unpleasant like rotten eggs, and gushed like a hydrant of water, were worse in the morning and occasionally involuntary. It was a hasty stool like you find in *Sulphur*, the patient had to run; there was a great deal of flatulence which was extremely foetid. Indeed the whole patient was offensive, the breath was terrible, as if it came straight out of a cesspool, the dry tongue was coated with a brownish fur. It recalled the description of *Psorinum* to me and after some twenty-four hours on *Arsenic*, on due consideration, I gave *Psorinum 9m,* the only potency available. I was badly hampered, as I was miles away from hospitals, from druggists and in a foreign country; the small village shops did not stock anything useful. A starch enema for the continual urging and pain and burning in the intestines would have helped, but there were no enema syringes to be had, and no starch. The only food offered as suitable for an invalid suffering from diarrhoea was rice water! Unfortunately the patient's stomach revolted at the idea of rice water and returned it promptly. Nobody had heard of arrowroot, and cornflour was unknown. Cranberries did grow on the slopes of the mountain side; but they were not ripe enough and not ready for use. Cranberry juice contains tannin and is first-rate for diarrhoea. Cranberries and bilberries either dried or freshly gathered when in season, should be soaked, if dried, and cooked until soft with a little sugar; then sieved and eaten with a dry rusk or toast.

There were no adjuvants to be had, only the homoeopathic remedy, so I gave *Psorinum 9m*, four hourly. Did this high potency act? These infinitesimal doses? It certainly did. The patient will confirm it if asked about it. She responded rapidly; it was not coincidence; she had been getting rapidly weaker and worse before the *Psorinum* was given; she only lived on sips of water, and had no other treatment except a few doses of the homoeopathic remedy. Three days after the attack of dysentry she was back in the hotel dining room, enjoying a good square meal which relieved the terrible weakness and exhaustion. She looked pale and drawn and more like a ghost, a mere shadow of her former self; but she was alive and able to digest her food. It was curious how quickly the offensive odour disappeared after the *Psorinum* was given.

After her return to England, the worst complaint was the anaemia, weakness and debility after the acute attack of diarrhoea and vomiting: and this was treated and disappeared within a short time after a few doses of no less a medicine than *Pulsatilla*! This brought back the desire to eat, the enjoyment of her food, and fattened the cheeks and removed the pallor and the weakness. Why was *Pulsatilla* given? It was noticed that the patient suffered from extreme heat and burning of the feet, so hot and burning they were thrust out of bed to cool (*Medorrhinum, Puls., Sulph.*). The patient was depressed and weepy, refused fat, complained of nausea after rich food; and she liked to be made a fuss of. *Pulsatilla* 30, and later 1*m* rapidly improved the remaining symptoms and restored a useful member of the community to health and strength. Homoeopathy works rapidly, too. This was a severe attack of diarrhoea and vomiting, as severe a one as I have ever seen in an adult; and yet the patient was up and about and there was no return after three days' treatment. The other patients in the Swiss Hotel who had the same complaint were in bed for over a week.

See how rapid the turnover in a hospital would be if the patients were treated homoeopathically in acute diseases. I am quite sure we should not want so many hospitals; there would not be such long waiting lists, the taxpayers' money would be saved and Industry would benefit, as there would be less sickness.

CHAPTER THREE

ANIMAL RESPONSE TO
HOMOEOPATHIC REMEDIES

'Our Tim' has gone to the Elysian Fields and I am not
ashamed to confess that I shed a few bitter tears when the
time came for parting with him. He had been ailing for seven
months from an affection of the liver which gradually and
relentlessly wore him down. All the same it was interesting to
watch how he responded to each remedy given on the
symptoms. He suffered from painless, sudden attacks of
diarrhoea, pale, almost white, liquid motions: aversion to fat,
he preferred skimmed milk to cream, for example; he
preferred to lie flat on his abdomen, as if pressure relieved
him; lack of appetite, he would start as if he enjoyed his food
and then leave off almost immediately, as if he was too full
already; and all his symptoms were worse every other day.
For this he had *China* in various potencies which usually
worked for 4-5 days, when he required another dose. This
carried him on for months, with an occasional dose of
Pulsatilla, as he became very affectionate and liked to be
petted, which was quite foreign to him; he was usually very
aloof and haughty and preferred to be left alone. It was very
instructive to see how *China* cleared up the diarrhoea for
days and gave him an appetite.

I kept on hoping that it would cure him, but it only acted
as a palliative and did not touch the disease. He was too old,
well over thirteen years of age, and there was no recuperative
power. He became thinner and thinner, and in the end we
decided it would be the kindest thing to part with him. But
Homoeopathy eased his sufferings, prolonged his life and
kept him happy until the last minute.

Homoeopathy does this always, even with humans; if the
span of life is nearly finished, and there is no deep-going
response to the remedies, when vitality is exhausted and

reaction fails, then our remedies still help and gradually the patient sinks without pain; it is then just a dissolution of the life forces. We do not require any morphia or other pain-killing drugs which cloud perception and dull the intelligence, and man, the soul and spirit of man is awake and active until the moment of death, when the silver cord is loosed, in the words of the Holy Bible.

All the same Homoeopathy reduces the death rate, as I have proved to my own satisfaction and shown it to others, over and over again.

Quite a brilliant example of this happened years ago. I was visiting a poor widow's family, who in spite of living in London had a great affection for country pursuits and kept all sorts of animals. She also kept poultry in her back garden and reared chickens successfully. Unfortunately at the time of my visits, the weather had turned very cold and damp; it was early April, and it was too cold for the newly hatched chickens, so they were brought in to the warmth and disported themselves on the large table in the parlour. All the same they did not thrive; one after the other died. They staggered round and round the table and were found dead.

I know next to nothing about chickens and their ailments; but restlessness and damp cold weather, I thought, meant *Rhus tox.*, so I gave *Rhus tox.* 30 to two of the chickens by opening their beaks, also putting more *Rhus tox.* into their water; these two chickens were the only ones which survived out of a brood of thirteen eggs. Coincidence, of course!

Another time a friend of mine was very perturbed about her canary who was moulting severely. He was moping, looked very pale, would not eat and would suddenly fall down off his perch and lie in his cage with his feet in the air, as if dead. The Vet called it heart-trouble and would not give a favourable diagnosis. I never saw the bird, but on these symptoms I sent one dose of *Sulphur* 6 and a few 2 grain pills of *Carbo veg.* 3x and *Nux vom.* 3x combined. The *Sulphur* was to be given first as a constitutional and half a pill of the *Carbo veg.* and *Nux vom.* was crushed and put in his drinking water, which was changed daily. The canary picked up at once; there were no further faints, if they were faints; he soon sported a beautiful coat of feathers and started to sing with renewed vigour.

The year after, at the next moult, these symptoms recurred, but not so severely and a few doses of *Carbo veg.* and *Nux vom.* with one dose of *Sulphur* again cut short the canary's misery.

The Vet. could not do anything; but a few doses of the homoeopathic remedies had the desired effect.

'Pooh — imagination, fiddlesticks,' I hear the disbelieving say. It was not due to faith on the animal's part, that it recovered, canaries have been known to die during a moult, and this canary recovered as soon as he was given these medicines. So why not give the credit to the medicines?

Still another pretty little tale about a lamb this time. The head of an agricultural college in Ireland who was the observer and whose permission I have to record it, noticed that one of the ewes refused to allow her newly-born lamb to suck. Ewes recognize their offspring by smell and refuse to nurse strange lambs. Once in a while a mother ewe will disown her baby and then the wee lamb will die soon, unless it is hand-fed with a bottle which is difficult and not always successful. My friend, who is a keen, knowledgeable lay homoeopath, pondered this problem of the ewe who did not have the usual mother instincts of an animal; then he recalled the proving of *Sepia*, where it says that hatred of and aversion to the loved one was a symptom brought out in the proving. He promptly went to his medicine case and gave the ewe some *Sepia*. By the next day the refractory mother ewe had forgotten its dislike to its little lamb and allowed it to nurse. And the lamb throve and grew big on its mother's milk. I understand, once a ewe refuses to nurse its lamb, it will never change its mind. Here the homoeopathic remedy once again worked according to rule.

There is much talk these days about foot and mouth disease in pigs and cattle; many thousands of useful dairy cattle are slaughtered and burnt on huge pyres to prevent the spread of this disease. Millions of pounds of money have been spent in compensating the farmers for the loss of their pigs and their cattle, and meanwhile the price of milk and butter is going up. All this could be saved if Homoeopathy were used for treating these cattle. They could be cured quickly, I am sure, with *Antimonium crudum*, which has the blisters on the tongue, thick white-coated tongue, bleeding of the gums and teeth, and cracks of the toes and red swellings of the heel; or with *Graphites*, which has vesicles and ulcers on the tongue, profuse salivation, and foetid sweat of the feet, ulceration of the toes, excoriation and sores between the toes. Just to mention two of the remedies which have some of the symptoms of foot and mouth disease. The animals would be cured quickly; there would be little fear of spread of infection; and the disease would die out quickly. I should imagine, too, that the different varieties of artificial manures which are used on grasslands have a great deal to do with animal disease. It is a pity as I have said before, that there are so few homoeopathic veterinary surgeons. The present-day vets know very little about treatment; they only seem to be slaughterers and do nothing but condemn the poor beasts to a premature death. Unfortunately the law of the land, as it stands at present, puts all the power into the hands of these ignorant men — ignorant as far as treatment is concerned; ignorant and biassed. A nosode from the secretion of the mouth and the discharging ulcers of the toes given in the 30th or 200th potency would cure this trouble even more rapidly. Dr. Darlington, a well-known agricultural scientist is reported to have said that the policy of the Ministry of Agriculture with regard to Foot and Mouth Disease is not only wasting hundreds of tons of prime beef every year, and by destroying every herd of cattle as soon as there is any sign of Foot and Mouth Disease in a particular herd, Britain is also losing the chance of building up herds immune to this disease. Therefore taxpayers' money is being wasted and food which is badly wanted in this time of universal shortage, is lost unnecessarily. This doctor believes that by applying discoveries already made the Ministry could increase very quickly the nation's home-produced food supplies, which sounds feasible. In his opinion the agricultural Research Council acts as a donkey cart driven by a blind man!

Homoeopathy is waiting to be discovered; the books are there, the knowledge is there, and it is only the blindness and the prejudice of the so-called scientific folk who will not even study it or try it out which prevents the *benefits of Homoeopathy* from being made known so that it can be used for suffering mankind and the Animal Kingdom.

CHAPTER FOUR

RESPIRATORY DISEASES

Bronchial Asthma is due to spasms of the bronchial muscles and it is closely related to hay fever which frequently alternates with asthma, so that the same patient may have asthma in the winter and hay fever in the early summer. These paroxysmal attacks of asthma and hay fever usually occur in families suffering from an irritable or unstable nervous system. One of its peculiarities is the extraordinary variety of circumstances which may induce a paroxysm: a patient may be free from attacks living in a house on one side of the road and may be put *hors de combat* by moving to a house exactly opposite. He may be free in the city and invariably suffer from attacks on going to a special part of the country. Emanations from animals, such as the horse or cat or dog, or odours of flowers or hay may at once cause an outbreak. Diet most certainly has a great influence and severe paroxysms may be brought on by overloading the stomach.

Affections of the nose such as hypertrophic rhinitis and nasal polypi are frequently associated with asthma.

Many and varied are the treatments suggested for the 'cure' of asthma. The greater the number of 'cures' vaunted the more difficult the cure, one usually finds. Asthma cures are the Happy Hunting Grounds of the quack vendor. There is the certain cure recommended by a long dead specialist who would turn in his grave if he knew to what use his name is put. The press and many magazines are full of advertisements for self-styled asthma treatments. What a harvest they must make, judging from the remarks of various patients one has come across. Each one has a different cure which is invariably the best, and the unfortunate victim has to go on using it — year in, year out. One extremely excitable individual one knew lived on iron jelloids all the year round, varied by somebody's pink pills for other ills whenever there was the slightest sign of breathlessness. During one fairly severe attack she was treated successfully and the duration was shortened considerably to two days instead of the usual week by four-hourly doses of *Carbo veg.* 30; and yet after it was over, she went back to iron jelloids and was rather annoyed than otherwise for getting well so quickly. She preferred the excitement of being ill and being the centre of interest to being made well rapidly. Smoking asthma cigarettes and making the whole household rush round after her getting the 'Cure' was more gratifying to her than lying quietly and taking small doses of inoffensive looking pilules — it was not dramatic enough. She was a typical example of a spoilt only daughter who could produce fainting attacks and asthma almost at will, and years afterwards when she had left this country, one still heard of her going on the same way, now playing up her poor husband instead of her parents by frequent attacks of asthma.

Some time ago while paying a visit to an asthma patient, one saw a table six feet by three feet long standing by the bedside laden with bottles and boxes and jars of all sizes and colours. She informed me that this was her medicine chest, all the things that she herself had bought or that her friends had sent her to cure her asthma. There were a dozen or more eight ounce bottles of various cough cures, syrups and cough linctus; there were several inhalers, Friar's Balsam and other balsams; several nasal sprays; and menthol mixtures for sprays, pinoleum and other pine mixtures for the same purpose; nasal ointments by the dozen; iodines, colourless and coloured, several jars for poultices. Various herbal mixtures for smoking, asthma cigarettes by the dozen; quite eight or ten patented cures, some came from Scotland, some from France, some from Germany. There were different medicated wools, yards of it. There were all kinds of boxes of pills. The only thing I did not see were leeches, by which another asthma patient swore; she had spent a great deal of time in France and the French doctors always applied these to various parts of her body, with, as far as I could hear, very little apparent result. I rather horrified the economically minded lady with her table full of potions when I suggested that she should throw the lot away into the dustbin, that we should not want any of them — nor did we.

In a very few weeks we had the lady sleeping well and naturally, without any Dial or Veronal, she required no further constipation tablets, the bronchitis had disappeared and the asthma was no more. *Coffea* 6 nightly made her sleep and a course of *Agaricus* in various potencies scotched the bronchitis and asthma. Now she sleeps soundly and has forgotten she ever had asthma. I don't think this was genuine asthma; I think it was brought on and aggravated by asthma cures, and once all these different medicines were thrown away, the patient got well.

Why was *Agaricus* given? It is not a medicine often thought of in chest troubles and yet it does cure bronchitis and asthma in the person who presents *Agaricus* symptoms. The *Agaricus* patient is usually a slender, willowy, nervous, restless person full of twitches, full of quiverings of muscles, tingling of nerves, clumsy, awkward, falling about, dropping things continually and breaking them, feeling the cold intensely, with a tendency to consumption, there are coughing fits ending in sneezes. Bad nights, always full of great nervous irritation and instability. Violent coughing fits ending in sneezes. Bad nights from breathlessness, palpitations, jerking of limbs followed by extreme tiredness and weariness in the morning, but towards evening the patient brightens up and is full of cheer and able to do things. *Agaricus* takes hold of such a person, and in time, perhaps it may take months, it will alter the whole outlook and the whole constitution. Many years ago, during the 1914-18 war, one came across another asthma patient. She was also tall and thin, with a greasy skin, pallid, lackadaisical, emphysematous chest and a history of bronchitis and asthma for eighteen years since the age of fourteen. About two or three months before her first attack of asthma she had been vaccinated for the first time. I fancy there was a small-pox scare on at the time. She certainly escaped small-pox, but fell a victim to bronchitis and asthma instead. For years she had been treated both as an in- and out-patient at one of the larger teaching hospitals with no improvement. The history seemed plain, asthma following shortly after vaccination, her face was pallid, sickly, waxy and shiny, her hands were horny and split open frequently, she had had warts off and on. She felt the cold intensely and suffered much from indigestion, specially after drinking tea. *Thuja* 30 was given and she was kept on *Thuja* 30 which was later on raised to *Thuja* m and *Thuja* 10*m* and the asthma was marvellously improved and the chest symptoms cleared up. She had one acute attack of asthma during the whole five years she was kept under observation, for which she was given *Puls.* 30 four hourly, and she had a dry teasing cough, which was worse lying down, she wanted the windows open, had a great desire for fresh air, she was weepy and tearful, wanted a lot of sympathy and the bronchial chill had come on after getting her feet wet. What else could this be but *Pulsatilla?* and *Puls.* 30 cured rapidly. As I said, for five years she kept well and then she moved away. One tried to persuade her to keep under a homoeopathic doctor. She acknowledged that she had never felt so well and that she was a totally different person since she had had the treatment. Yet she fell into the hands of the Philistines, was given various serum and other injections at the next attack and some three or four years later she died of asthma and heart. The more is the pity thereof.

Some years ago a Mrs. H. was persuaded to come to the dispensary to get relief from asthma. She was not at all sure that anything could be done for her. She had been an in-patient at a nearby General Hospital for months, she had asthma, she had heart trouble and nothing could cure her, the doctors at the ''ospital' had told her so. She was a big stout coster-woman, highly-coloured face, puffing and panting, hardly able to crawl along, cyanosed cheeks, bluish lips and very fond of her glass of stout. Not a very promising case. For her immediate distress she was given *Arsenic* 6, which was prescribed, because her asthma always came on about

midnight or shortly after, was worse between 12 a.m. and
2 a.m. She was restless, full of agitating fears, very weak and
prostrated and always had a craving for warm drinks or sips
of hot water which relieved her breathlessness. Jahr. in his
Manual of Forty Years' Practice always advises the doctor to
start all acute cases of asthma on either *Arsenic* or
Ipecacuanha according to the symptoms. Here the symptoms
called for *Arsenic* and *Arsenic* was given as a preliminary.
One wondered whether really much could be done for such a
case who had been ill for years. In a week she came back full
of praise for the marvellous powders she had had. She had
never felt such rapid relief and the bronchitis was so much
better. She was given further doses of *Ars.* 6 and was not seen
again for nearly fifteen months. She had kept these miraculous powders safely and had only taken an occasional dose at
night when an attack had threatened to come on and there
had been none now for nearly twelve months. This is the
right method of treating and curing any acute illness; *take the
medicine while ill, leave off when feeling better and resume
the treatment when the symptoms recur.* This time she had
another severe attack, and as she had no more powders, she
came for a repeat. She looked so blue, so cyanosed, that very
foolishly one gave her *Lachesis* 30, as she was awakened out
of her sleep by attacks of asthma. She came back the next
week, very hurt, 'these were not the same powders, they had
not done her any good. She wanted the old powders'. She
was quite right as it turned out. So once again she was given
twelve powders of *Arsenic* 6 with the same miraculous result!
One did not see her very often after that, she would
occasionally send for a repeat, she liked to keep them at hand
in case of need. The asthma and heart promptly disappeared
again, she has had no return of the asthma for several years
now, in her case the *Ars.* was not only her acute remedy, but
acted as the chronic medicine. It prevented the asthmatical
attacks and aborted them so satisfactorily that for years she
has been free, much to her husband's relief, who suffered
much from her restlessness and her nightly fits of coughing.
This typical coster-woman still loves her glass, still has her

occasional booze and is very much feared for her virulent tongue and her stout fists in the occasional brawls in the local alley where she lives, but there is no more asthma.

Not all asthma cases are as easy to relieve or cure as this one was. Some cases require years of treatment and some require to be kept under observation for many months, and even though they may require almost continuous treatment, the relief is more lasting and the damage to the heart and lungs is less than if orthodox treatment were given. One can keep the asthma at bay with the homoeopathic remedies so much more easily than the usual much vaunted cures, which undermine a patient's health.

Mrs. H's asthma, so easily cured by *Ars.*, was what Hahnemann calls a psoric manifestation of her constitution and, therefore, a psoric such as *Ars.* cured so quickly. Most cases of asthma are, however, complicated by sycosis and then you require sycotic medicines, and it takes years to rout the enemy and much careful prescribing before the patient is on the road to health.

Natrum sulph. is a very common remedy, often required to relieve asthma in such a wet climate as ours. One busy morning at the dispensary I was called to see an acute case of asthma who had alarmed the efficient caretaker very much. There was not time to go into great details, one just noticed that she always had an attack when it was wet and warm. On this indication she was given *Nat. Sulph.* 30 with prompt disappearance of her trouble. She kept free for two or three months, and then the action had worked out and whenever the weather turned wet and rainy on came another attack. She usually required treatment every three or four months, then came a long spell of freedom for nearly two years and then a return of her trouble, she was given *Nat. sulph. m* which again helped for three months, even though the weather remained wet she would not want a repetition for several months. She might forget to come and put up with the asthma for a week or so, but as soon as she was given a dose of *Nat. sulph.* the attacks stopped. Unfortunately she lived so near the borderline of starvation and poverty that very little permanent good could be done for her.

In the *Nat. sulph.* patient the asthma usually comes on later than in an *Ars.* patient, the asthma attack does not start until 4 a.m. or 5 a.m. and lasts through the fore-noon. It has a loose humid cough with copious viscid greenish-yellow phlegm; the chest feels sore and oppressed and holding the chest with the hand relieves the cough. *Nat. sulph.* often follows after *Ars.* has relieved the acute attack, and it is often a complement and follows well after *Thuja*, when *Thuja* fails to relieve; but again in some cases *Nat. sulph.* ceases to hold the patient and one wants another sycotic remedy, which goes deeper, and frequently *Medorrhinum* takes up the case and finishes it.

It is no wonder in these days of excessive speed, nauseous petrol fumes, raucous gramophones and blaring loudspeakers that children who are 'belasted' as the Germans so graphically describe it, who are weighed down or heavily burdened by an unstable nervous system, should show early signs of asthma, which is a typical nervous affliction of the respiratory apparatus. A sequence of events as the following has been noted several times: healthy father, badly gassed in the war, marrying an excitable French woman who had many harrowing experiences during the war, the offspring developed asthma at the early age of four. Or a very powerful personality, full of alarms and excursions, always either in the depths of despair or right up in the clouds with joy, supersensitive to everything, excitable; in her acute ailments always a typical *Belladonna* case, passed on this unstable, nervous temperament to her grandson in whom it became accentuated and broke out as recurrent asthmatic attacks with each slight cold: which showed first during the dentition period, before he was a year old. The child was never coddled, always kept very spartan and hardened as much as possible, had a daily cold sponging down, never wore a hat, winter or summer, and yet always these nervous explosions, bronchitis with each cold and asthma, and even frequent broncho-pneumonias. He was given *Hepar sulph.* 6 and kept on it, as he apparently always developed asthma following an

exposure to a cold, dry, east wind. It did not prevent the
attacks, it modified them slightly; he would be ill for four or
five days instead of two or three weeks. Still it went on, year
after year, exposure to wind, an acute attack the next night,
ill in bed for several days. At the age of seven he was taken to
the seaside, the South Coast, for the summer and improved at
once, no attack for the whole two months he was there.

On this symptom, improvement at the seaside, worse cold
wind, he was given *Medorrhinum* 30 and now for eight
months he has been quite free from bronchitis and asthma;
all through the winter he attended school regularly in all
kinds of weather! He will want an occasional course of
Medorrhinum for several years. Asthma in young children
requires in my experience at least two and a half to three or
four years treatment, before this tendency to asthma is
completely eradicated. It is worth while, isn't it, to stop these
harassing experiences, harassing to the parents and alarming
to the child, as these awful spasms of the chest muscles are?

The Anglo-French boy I mentioned previously was first
seen in 1930 when he was nine years old, undersized, with
stooping shoulders, pigeon-chested, with retracted ribs, no
expansion of the lower half of the chest muscles, excessive
movements of the accessory respiratory muscles of the neck,
cyanosed lips and bluish cheeks, gasping and panting, shallow
breathing. Had these attacks for years. He was put in the
Physical Therapy Department of the Dispensary where he
had bi-weekly treatment — breathing exercises to expand his
chest muscles and to oxygenate his lungs; general exercises to
improve his physique, radiant light with the Murray Levick
lamp and three minutes each on front and back of the trunk
with the cold Mercury Vapour lamp. His physique improved,
slowly, but the asthma did not. Then there was almost a
catastrophe. On the advice of a well-meaning, interfering
busy-body of a voluntary lady-visitor who goes round
pestering the lives of our poor by offering gratuitous advice
to them and interfering freely with the business of the
trained health workers — doctors and nurses — the mother
was persuaded to send this delicate boy, who was carefully

watched and guarded at home against draughts, to a fortnightly open-air camp in order to harden him! It was a cold wet July and the boy promptly developed pneumonia and nearly died. When I saw him next, two months later, the work of six months treatment was spoilt and we had to start right from the beginning again: mild exercises, gradually increasing in severity, light, etc. A few months later, in November, 1931, he was given his first course of Homoeopathy. It was observed that he was always chilly, always catching colds, very easily tired and exhausted, especially in the afternoon between 4 and 8 o'clock. He was a timid, shy lad, whenever he developed a cold it would fly at once to his chest and after a week of right-sided lung trouble it would extend to the left side. All typical *Lycopodium* symptoms, and he was kept on infrequent doses of *Lyc*. 30. The improvement was apparent at once, the attacks of asthma came on less and less often.

At the fortnightly visits the reports always were from now on: no bronchitis, no breathlessness, clear breath-sounds. For ten months he was free of asthma, until September, 1932, when he caught a cold and continued catching colds for the next four weeks, yet there was no asthma; *Lyc*. given on October 6th, 1932. November 24th, 1932, again *Lyc*. was given, as there was still a weakened resistance to colds. February 6th, 1933, no asthma, no colds for months, has not been attending for 'light' treatment or physical exercises since early December, 1932, does not think it is necessary, as he feels so well now. *Lyc*. 30 given (February 9th, 1933). Not seen again until November 15th, 1934, when he had another cold; chest well developed now, sturdy lad, no emphysema, no bronchitis for months, *Lyc*. 30. In November, 1934, he was nearly fourteen, at school leaving age, and he promised to attend whenever his chest troubled him. Not seen again until the summer, 1936, when he called to report that he was getting on splendidly.

He is now a young man nearly 5 feet 10 inches in height, has a broad and massive chest, is quite unrecognizable, a totally different proposition from the puny, ill-looking, panting boy of six years ago. Is Homoeopathy worth while? Light and exercise are good auxiliary measures in asthma, but they are disappointing by themselves. This lad attended regularly bi-weekly for months, and yet there were constant reports of bronchitis, attacks of breathlessness, asthma and so on until November, 1931, when he had his first dose of homoeopathic medicine, *Lyc.*, which corresponded to his symptoms, and then the attacks ceased almost at once and he became irregular in his attendances, as he was so well. The exercises and light helped his physical development, but the most marked improvement came on after the *Lyc.* and he began to grow in stature and in weight. On sending an enquiry to his home address a few weeks ago, I was informed that he had no further asthma! What a different existence it would have been for this lad, if he had not been given homoeopathic treatment. And how many there are like him, a drag on the labour market, delicate, puny, unable to pull their weight, and always collapsing at the wrong moment. It is not so serious when you have a private income of your own or earn sufficiently to be able to stand the expense of recurrent enforced holidays, made necessary by asthma, but to the wage-earner with a small weekly wage, asthma is a very serious enemy. And Homoeopathy can and does deal with it satisfactorily. In some cases, especially in young folk, it eradicates the complaint entirely. In others, in older people, it makes life much more possible, it shortens the attacks and may even prevent them. But it may need prolonged treatment and careful, very careful medication.

F.R. Boy aged twelve. Seen September 1st, 1932, recurrent attacks of bronchitis and asthma. Had asthma for years with typical deformity of chest. Light and exercises advised, attended regularly at the Physical Exercises Department, was watched carefully for three months. It was impossible to get many symptoms from him, he was too vague. Then it was noticed that the attacks were worse during damp weather, he was always taking colds during wet, rainy weather; on this symptom one gave him *Nat. sulph. m*, on December 21st, 1932, and to one's joy it acted well. He had no attacks until

May 4th, 1933, when he caught his first cold due to getting wet, which developed into bronchitis and asthma. On May 25th, 1933, he had another course of *Nat. sulph. m*, no asthma then until March, 1934; he was free for ten months: all through summer and autumn and even the winter of 1933-34 — a record! *Nat. sulph. m* was given again on March 15th, 1934, and one heard during the summer of 1934 that he had kept well. Unfortunately one has lost sight of him since then, but during the eighteen months' treatment he had, he put on weight, lost his bronchitis and developed into a fine young lad, and the asthma became negligible and disappeared for months on end.

A.G., a lad aged eleven, first seen May, 1933. Had asthma for years since an attack of diphtheria at the age of three, has attended Brompton Hospital. On examination, emphysema, no expansion of chest, very slight movement of chest wall in an upward direction only, can raise phlegm with difficulty, does not like wet weather, vomits with cough. *Ipecac.* 30 t.d.s. June 8th, 1933, cough worse nights. Lungs: asthmatic sounds all over, *Ars.* 30 t.d.s. June 15th, 1933, no change though sleeping better at night, *Lyc.* 30, one dose and *Ipecac.* 30 t.d.s. for the asthma attacks.

June 22nd, 1933, deeply cyanosed lips and ears, breathing very laboured, asthmatic sounds all over, *Ipecac.* 30 t.d.s.

July 6th, lungs clear, no cough, but weekly attacks always on Sunday nights for several weeks, *Sulph.* 30 (one dose) and *Ipecac.* 30 t.d.s. for acute attacks.

July 20th, 1933, lungs, rhonchi and râles, still an acute attack on Sunday, not cyanosed this week, *Nat. sulph. m*, one dose, mainly on indication that he did not like wet weather.

September 7th, 1933. Very irritable before attacks come on; has had asthma ever since attack of diphtheria as a young child. *Thuja* 30 given mainly on the assumption that he probably had diphtheria anti-toxin in the fever hospital and *Thuja* is an antidote to anti-toxin inoculation.

September 21st, 1933. Bad attack last Sunday, very difficult boy, never speaks for himself, always accompanied by his mother, who is very unobservant, the lad himself is very bad tempered and irritable before an attack, otherwise he never complains. As one could get no very definite symptoms out of either the mother or the lad, one had to be content in giving the acute remedy in repeated doses, namely *Ipecac.* 30 t.d.s. week after week, which alleviated to a certain extent. Had no bad attacks until October 12th, when on the assumption that *Thuja* given on September 7th had kept him comparatively free of 'turns' and would probably help again, *Thuja* 30 was given again. *Ipecac.* 30 t.d.s. for the paroxysms.

November 2nd, 1933. Attack during night (between two and three o'clock), screams in sleep, fights with other children, lungs: sibili, very dry cough; *Tuberculin* 30 and *Ipecac* 30, t.d.s. for paroxysms.

November 9th, 1933, worse during fog, lungs clear, not so cyanosed, no screaming attacks; *Diphtherinum* 30 to antidote the diphtheria he had as an infant.

November 16th. Well all the week, even though it is foggy weather, does not like being home, easily frightened, never comes without his mother, never speaks up for himself. *Ipecac.* 30 t.d.s.

November 23rd, 1933. Bites nails, cannot stick fats, hangs on to mother's apron strings, never talks to strangers, lungs: sibili. *Puls.* 30 t.d.s. for three days.

November 30th, 1933. Very much better, weight 4 st. 11 lb., attacks come on early morning, 5 a.m.

Was kept on *Puls.* 30 in repeated doses during December, 1933, with the report: no wheezing now, constant wheezing last year during December.

January 25th, 1934. Bad attacks with wheezing and breathlessness during week-end. *Puls.* 30 t.d.s.

March 8th, 1934. Weight, 4 st. 13 lb., gain of two pounds in four months, cold during week, very thirsty, limbs ached all over, a few rhonchi and sibili. *Bry.* 30 t.d.s., kept on *Bry.* for the next few weeks.

March 22nd. No cyanosis now, no bad attacks during night, lungs: a little roughness at end of respiration. *Bry.* 30 t.d.s.

April 15th, 1934. Boil right leg, glands enlarged right groin. *Tarantula cubensis* 30, four doses. *Tarent. cub.* being almost a specific for boils.

April 25th. Weight 4 st. 10 lb. 12 oz., no cyanosis, no turns during night, no shortness of breath.

May 17th, 1934. Loose cough, lungs: a few scattered rhonchi. *Tarant. cub.* 30, three doses.

June 7th, 1934. Sits up in bed and chokes at 2 to 3 a.m., wants fresh air. *Ars.* 30 during paroxysms. Occasional doses of *Ars.* 30 given by mother, he only required one dose a week usually.

July 12th, 1934. Much better, no attacks, has been to Epsom on his bicycle by himself, never used to stir without his mother in the past. Kept on *Ars.* 30 when necessary during August and September, 1934. Weight 5 st.

September 20th, 1934. Face very blue again. Asthma < lying down. < during night, wakes him up, very warm during attack. *Lach.* 30. Worse during September and October. So bad that mother despaired of his ever getting well and took him off to Brompton Hospital, as she was afraid he had tuberculosis of the lungs. Reassured by hospital that, as he was having light treatment and physical exercises, he was having the best treatment for his complaint and advised to keep him under the dispensary. Mother returned with her tail between her legs, rather shamefaced for having gone elsewhere for advice. The hospital X-rayed him as well, found only asthma, no tuberculosis. Boy was very much worse while he was having medicinal treatment from the hospital during the last four weeks. In bed most of the time with acute paroxysms of cough and breathlessness. November 8th, 1934, *Lyc.* 30. Weight 4 st. 12 lb. 8 oz., lost a good deal of weight during the last six weeks.

December 13th, 1934. Sleeps well at night. Lungs, rhonchi only on the right side (*Lyc.* symptom) repeated *Lyc.* 30.

January 10th, 1935. No attacks since middle of December, no cyanosis, hardly any altered breath sounds.

January 24th, 1935. Shortness of breath worse 4 to 5 a.m., not so much asthma lately, worse during week-ends, lungs, rhonchi and rales right side. *Kali carb.* 30.

January 31st, 1935. Felt very tired after the powder last week, sleeping very well. Lungs, just a few dry sounds.

February 14th, 1935. No attacks since January 24th, early morning breathlessness nearly gone.

February 21st, 1935. Bad all day yesterday since 5 a.m. *Kali carb.* 30.

March 7th, 1935. Very well until yesterday (slight fog), a few whistling sibili in lungs. *Kali carb.* 30.

March 28th, 1935. Worse again Saturday and Sunday. Lungs, full of rhonchi. *Kali carb.* 30.

April 11th. Lungs full of rhonchi and râles worse 4 to 5 a.m. *Kali carb.* 30, three powders to be taken night and morning.

May 2nd. Much better, goes out more, likes playing out of doors now.

May 9th. Return of asthma at thought of going back to school. *Kali carb.* 30, three powders.

June 13th. Very much better until week-end (wet weather). *Kali carb.* 30.

July 12th, 1935. Plays cricket in school now, speaks up for himself, sleeps well.

September, 1935. Has been well for months, developed a wart on tip of the nose, which dropped off during holidays.

September 26th, 1935. Bad nights again. Lungs, sibili. *Kali carb.* 30.

October 3rd, 1935. No change. *Kali carb. m.*

October 10th. No asthma, but bad cold after fog, thirsty, dry cough, terribly irritable. *Bry.* 30, t.d.s. Continued well through the winter until January 23rd, 1936 (for over three months no asthma), when he developed a cold and required another dose of *Kali carb. m,* which was followed by great improvement of his general condition. His breath-sounds remained clear. His mental condition improved, he became more independent, came alone for treatment, went out by himself, until April 2nd when he went to the 'pictures' and had an attack of asthma during the night (*Kali carb. m*), well again until May 14th, 1936, when a severe paroxysm troubled him again. *Kali carb. m.*

May 28th. Very well, great mental improvement, much brighter and more intelligent.

June 11th, 1936, return of asthma. *Kali carb m.*

July 9th, 1936. Very well, no asthma, chest development good, chest expansion good, no deformity of chest muscles now. Discharged as he was now fourteen, and was going out to work. Seen, Spring, 1937, continues well, no asthma. Met him in the street early 1938. Asthma again. *Kali carb.*10*m* sent; no further treatment. Seen September 1941, in excellent condition, no breathless attacks, on regular work.

I have given this boy's case with great detail, as it was difficult to find the right constitutional remedy at first, his acute attacks were alleviated by acute remedies such as *Ipecac.* and *Ars.*, but in spite of faithful attendances at the physical therapy classes, where he had breathing exercises and light treatment, he continued to wheeze and continued to have attacks, until gradually I saw the picture of *Kali carb.*, and *Kali carb.* kept the attacks at bay and improved him mentally, psychologically and bodily as well. He, or rather his mother, got fed up in the middle of the treatment, as we were so slow in really curing him. Eventually at the end, she had to acknowledge that we had made a good job of him. *Kali carb.* is a difficult remedy to spot. It is sensitive to all atmospheric changes, draughts and colds, irritable and full of fears and imaginations. It is usually worse between 2 and 5 a.m., gets a cough with vomiting; this lad had cough with vomiting right until the time when he had *Kali carb.* which stopped the vomiting. His right side was more affected than the left side. It took a very long time to discover these symptoms, as they were a silent pair and only told you that he had an attack again, but were incapable of describing the attacks or giving full details, until gradually one had observed the symptoms for oneself. *Kali carb.* belongs to the sycotic range of medicines, and in asthma, chronic recurrent asthma, one usually has to find the suitable remedy among these sycotics, such as the *Kali* salts, *Medorrhinum, Nat. sulph., Staph., Sulph., Thuja*, and so on.

Asthma is a constitutional complaint and very often hereditary, and shows itself in various members of several generations; and asthma, when hereditary, is one of the 'sycotic complaints' of our Master, Hahnemann. I had a curious confirmation of this fact in one of the families I came across. The mother was a very delicate, pale, transparent-looking woman in the thirties, who had produced a large family of delicate children. With each pregnancy she became more and more waxy looking, more and more desperately ill, so ill that even hardened hospital authorities put her to bed for weeks beforehand and had her in the wards. This happened with three or four successive pregnancies. In between she recovered somewhat, even though she was always ailing, always out of breath, always anaemic — not exactly asthmatic, but always unable to drag about and always expected to die with each child, and yet always recovering. We got hold of her and gave her *Medorrhinum*, largely because the then infant had a characteristic ham-like eruption all over the buttocks and privates; this cleared up in a week after giving the mother *Medorrhinum* 30, and also giving the same medicine to the baby as well. We kept the baby on weekly doses of it, and lo and behold! it was the first baby that throve and got on and in due course became a bonny, strong child. The mother also suddenly started to put on weight, became less anaemic and more able to cope with her household duties and her numerous offspring. Then we heard that there was an older boy of six or so who had almost continuous attacks of asthma in the day-time, when he had to be rushed off to the local municipal hospital or the general teaching hospital, where he was usually kept in for several weeks at a time. He had just been away to the Isle of Wight for six months at a convalescent home; and I was told he had been simply splendid there and never had an attack the whole of the time, even though it was winter. Within two days of coming back to London there was another severe attack. Asthma during the day-time, asthma better at the seaside, and with a sycotic family history, the mother and brother doing well on *Med.*, we had the necessary tripod on

which to base our prescription. He was given *Med.* 30 and
kept on it for weeks, and it worked. The asthma attacks
ceased, he could attend school regularly, which he had not
done previously, and there was no further need for expensive
and prolonged convalescence in a seaside home. What a saving
to public and charitable funds!

There must be hundreds of such cases up and down the
country, who for the want of *Med.* continue to have asthma;
who are sent to the seaside or on long cruises in order to get
relief from this troublesome complaint. If only the knowledge of Homoeopathy would spread; one would like to
shout from the housetops: 'Go to a homoeopathic hospital or
doctor for your chronic, so-called incurable complaints, and
you will get relief, if not a cure; it may take time, it may take
a great deal of patience, but you will get it eventually.'

Talking about this symptom: 'relief of asthma at the
seaside', which points to *Med.*, there is another curious
symptom: 'Asthma of sailors as soon as they go ashore;
relieved again as soon as they are at sea.' This variety of
asthma is covered by *Bromine.* One remembers the case of a
fifty-year-old sea pilot, a big stout chap weighing 18 stones, a
fair-haired, blue-eyed man with apple-red cheeks. He was laid
up with asthma all the time he was on land and they thought
of pensioning him off, even though the moment he got on to
a ship he recovered. *Bromine* 6, three times a day, given for a
spell, made it possible for him to return to his job. If you
know this tip and many, many other *idiosyncrasies* of your
patients, they will enable you to cure diseases which are the
despair of the medical profession and even more so of the
individual who suffers.

Now to go back to proving our theory: that antisycotic
remedies cure asthma, and I mean *cure*, not just relieve!

A girl was seen in September, 1929, five years old who had
chest trouble for over twelve months, following on an attack
of broncho-pneumonia; she was ordered ultra-violet ray
treatment and exercises, which she carried out more or less
for two or three months; but the bronchial and asthmatic
attacks did not really diminish, and the family got tired of it

and took her to hospital. Five years later, on November 8th, 1934, she turned up again, having attended the local hospital during the whole of the time *with no result.* In the meantime they had heard of other cases of asthma who had been cured at our Dispensary, and thought they would try again what we could do.

She was a typical case of humid asthma: the chest was full of numerous mucous râles, rattling noises, and she was continually expectorating large quantities of white, thick, ropy mucus; there was a pain and an all-gone feeling in the chest, she had to hold it when she was coughing. The child presented a pitiful appearance, round shouldered, under-sized, thin, with kyphosis (curvature of spine), the ribs were drawn in, the upper part of the chest was barrel-shaped, her face was bluish. I found out that she was always worse in wet weather. All these symptoms pointed to *Nat. sulph.* and she was therefore given *Nat. sulph.* 30 and ordered to attend twice weekly for artificial sunlight and breathing exercises. A week later the report was: much better; and on examination the chest was found to be clear of abnormal sounds. November 22nd, 1934: 'bad during week, brings up a lot of phlegm; lungs clear.'

December 6th. Great deal of phlegm, lungs rattling — very wet and muggy weather; had been in bed for several days. *Nat. sulph.* 30, night and morning for three days.

December 13th. No bad breathing; eating better.

January 10th, 1935. In bed for three days just after Christmas, during rainy weather; attack was much shorter than usual; posture much improved. A few dry rhonchi found — no moist râles as before. *Nat. Sulph.* 30, one dose at once and then one dose to be given night and morning if a fresh attack developed.

January 24th. Very well; no attack and no *Nat. sulph.* required.

Remained free from attacks until February 14th. *Nat. sulph.* 30 (six doses), night and morning.

February 21st. Very wet weather, had been in bed for four days; profuse phlegm, yellowish-green and sticky — but attack not so severe as it used to be. *Nat. sulph.* 30 had worked out, as attacks came on more frequently and a higher potency was required, *Nat. sulph* 1m was given. Free from asthma until March 9th (a fortnight). Lungs however clear on the day she was examined. As I had no *Nat. sulph.* in the 1m potency at hand, I ordered again *Nat. sulph.* 30, twelve doses, night and morning, which kept her free from attacks for a whole month, and it was then repeated, twelve doses, three times a day during an attack.

May 2nd. Two attacks of a mild nature during week. *Nat. sulph.* 30 (twelve doses) when necessary. School doctor advised open-air school, but as she would miss her exercises and light treatment if she went to an open-air school, the mother was advised to refuse this offer of open-air treatment; also I did not think that open-air was very good for this kind of asthma, which came on during wet weather. She had to be kept continually on *Nat. sulph.* during the whole of the month of May, 1935. The attacks were milder and not so long lasting; they were relieved easily, but it seemed to me that *Nat. sulph.* was not going deep enough – another remedy was required.

On June 6th she reported that she had asthma every week for three weeks, running from Friday until Tuesday every week – and it was elicited that she 'lies in the knee-chest position with her face buried in the pillows during an attack'. This clearly pointed to *Med.*, and the medicine was changed to *Med.* 30. Kent, I think in his *Newer Remedies*, states that when *Nat. sulph.* does not seem to hold a case, the complementary medicine which goes deeper is *Med.*

June 20th, 1935. Another slight attack. *Med.* 30.

July 11th. No attacks for three weeks.

Weight: 4 st. 10 lb. 4 oz. She was then eleven years old, and the first time she was weighed at the Dispensary. Unfortunately it had been omitted to weigh her before, or, I am sure, she would have shown a considerable increase in weight, as she looked so much better and happier, and her attendance at school was much more regular.

September 26th, 1935. NO ATTACKS OF ASTHMA FOR

THREE MONTHS, not since June 20th; the very first time in her life that she had been free from her curse for such a long period. She had a very mild attack, and was only in bed for half-a-day (the middle of September) when the mother had given her a dose of *Med.* 30, which she had been told to do in an emergency. Report: limbs much stronger, no retraction of ribs.

October 3rd. *No attacks,* even though the *weather is wet and stormy.* You see how the right remedy alters the whole make-up of a person. She can now stand even wet weather, which she never could before.

October 17th, 1935. Attack during week; lies again on her face with the buttocks uppermost, all curled up. *Med.* 30.

October 31st. Coughs more during day-time; attacks during day-time; lies in knee-chest position. *Med.* 1*m*, which was repeated on November 14th and December 12th.

January 9th, 1936. Slight attack. *Med.* 2*m*. A slightly higher potency seemed to be required — no attacks until

February 6th (one month). *Med.* 30 (three doses), as she was sleeping on her face again.

February 27th. Slight attack. *Med.* 30, every night. March 5th. Very bad during week. Asthma bad during daytime. *Placebo.*

March 26. Slight attack. Repeat night and morning.

April 20th. Sleeps on face. Attacks only during daytime. *Med.* 30 every morning.

May 21st. First attack for three weeks. *Med.* 1*m*.

September 3rd. No attack since May 21st. Free for 3½ months now.

Weight is 5 st. 7 lb. — a gain of 11 lb. since July, 1935, i.e. in fourteen months. One would hardly know her as the same child. Chest expansion 3 ins. There was no expansion of chest at all when she was first taken in hand in November, 1934. No medicine since May 21st, 1936, for 3½ months.

October 8th, 1936. Slight attack after a chill. *Med.* 1*m*.

October 22nd. Weight 5 st. 10 lb. — gain 3 lb. in six weeks.

December 3rd. No attack since October 8th.

Weight 5 st. 12 lb. 4 oz. — gain of 2¼ lb. in six weeks, it is positively alarming how she puts on weight.

December 17th. Had a dose of *Med.* 1*m* during week, as she did not seem so well and the attack did not materialize; only one attack of asthma in seven months, and that only a mild one.

February 18th, 1937. Mild attack; sleeps again on her knees and chest. Mother says, she knows an attack is coming, when she finds her sleeping on her knees and chest, with the buttocks stuck out uppermost. *Med.* 1*m*, six doses to be given nightly.

March 4th. Attack again; feels cold, is very restless during night. *Arsenicum* 30, four hourly.

March 18th. Bad attack again. A higher potency of *Med.* is required, as attacks are more frequent again. (*Med.* 10*m*, to be given when necessary.)

April 8th. Weight 6 st. 2 lb.; still gaining weight; has not had *Med.* 10*m* yet.

May 6th. Another attack. *Med.* 10*m* given by mother.

May 20th, 1937. Weight 6 st. 3 lb. 8 oz. This child has gained 1½ stones in weight in not quite two years; the attacks of asthma are of rare occurrence and of short duration and only very mild — instead of being almost continuous and very severe. She is enjoying school, has grown into a big, pretty girl, and will be of some use in this world and able to earn her own living in the future, instead of being an expense to her family, and probably also to the ratepayers, as she would have to be always under hospital and have long spells of in-patient treatment. What a different life she would have led, if she had not been introduced to Homoeopathy. Her mother and her family swear by our treatment, and, in fact, swear by the powders; they were taught to give the emergency powders only when needed during an attack or when an attack was threatening; and they carried it out faithfully. *Med.* is a nosode, a remedy which only requires to be repeated at rare intervals; or you would get serious aggravations. Met her unexpectedly in August, 1941; did not know her until she introduced herself, she had grown into such a bonny young woman, in steady work, enjoying life. Has grown out of asthma 'with the help of Homoeopathy'. No attacks since the last dose in May 1937.

She broke down again in the winter of 1944, after she had been free of asthma for seven years. She developed pleurisy first, then gradually asthma reappeared; being under the panel doctor, she got steadily worse for 12 months. Eventually she came back to me, and within four weeks she was back at work, cured of her asthma again with *Med.* 10*m*.

You see from this case that asthma requires careful prescribing and it takes some years to combat this inherited tendency; but what a difference it makes. What a joy it is to see a child grow up from being a stunted, miserable being into a pretty, healthy and useful member of society. Can the Old School of Medicine do the same with the asthma cases under their care? I have seen no reports of progress made with their serums, their inoculations. The attacks usually seem to continue with the same severity year in, year out. They can tell you what brings on the attack, cat's hair, or effluvia from horses, certain kinds of articles of food; and the people are advised to keep away from horses or from cats, and give up eating eggs or whatever else may bring on an attack. Very tiresome to keep away from horses, should you be a jockey or an agricultural labourer. How much better to cure the tendency to asthma by the appropriate remedy and you will be able to live with a dozen cats in your home, and sleep in a stable full of horses. When will the profession learn to treat their patients rationally?

Is Asthma really curable? I have made a definite assertion that it is, and I have tried to show you by giving you the history of some cases seen and treated, that asthma yields to the indicated remedy. Now let us see what other authorities say about it. Dr. Kent in one of his later books states that for years he considered that asthma could be relieved; each attack could be cleared up by the indicated acute remedy. Some cases would show *Ipecac.* symptoms and *Ipecac.* would help quickly: others were definitely *Ars.* and *Ars.* in repeated doses cut the attack short. Others responded to *Spongia* and so on. But the enemy was not definitely thrown out, it still lurked in the background and would attack the unfortunate victim again and again. But Kent, being a genius, would not give in easily and studied his case most carefully and then the light came to him; there was a constitutional defect behind it all or a miasm as Hahnemann calls it graphically. It was not due to Psora, that is the constitutional disease imparted to the human organism in successive generations after the itch icarus had been suppressed by means of strong ointments. Itch was very prevalent a few centuries ago and was effectively driven in by the then medical pundits by strong unguents and lotions; and the evil effect showed itself in the children and children's children. But there are other constitutional defects, there is syphilis, brought to Europe after the discovery of America, but syphilitic remedies did not cure asthma always. Eventually, by a process of exclusion, Kent came to the conclusion that asthma was largely due to hidden sycosis: and that outside of sycotics you will seldom find a remedy for asthma. Sycosis is a constitutional defect or miasm, and is a product of animal toxins, introduced into the human body and foreign to it, such as smallpox, vaccination, gonorrhoea and I think and suspect strongly we shall get the same effects in the future from the many serums and inoculations now used. The sycotic state produces warts, cauliflower excrescences in the female, polypi and certain skin eruptions with definite peculiarities, and asthma which frequently alternates with skin troubles. I had an old lady many years ago who had this type of asthma, see-sawing between breathless attacks and a very ugly eruption on her hands and wrists. She was not content to let me treat this by medicine, she would put a proprietary ointment on her wrists so as to drive in her skin trouble and back would come the asthma. I pointed out gently that she was doing herself a great deal of harm. She was a sweet old lady, smiling placidly and happily through the worst attacks of asthma; *Mezereum* was her remedy — another sycotic medicine — but alas a *Mez.* eruption is a very uncomfortable one and she would not put up with it. A year or so later she came back with cauliflower growths on her external privates which were excessively painful. Alas! the sycosis that had been driven in had revenged itself and had become malignant. Nothing could be done for her, and I watched her slowly getting worse and worse, until she died in the local Infirmary. That was the first case in which it dawned on me that asthma and sycosis were closely related; later on I came across the family I mentioned previously where one member had a sycotic eruption on the buttocks, the older boy had asthma and the mother had sycotic anaemia and cardiac weaknesss. By the by, I heard yesterday that the mother is now so well that she is out at work all day besides looking after the family; which shows how well a woman who was thought to be dying can get on, if she gets the correct remedy — in this instance *Med.*

Med. is the homoeopathic nosode or vaccine made from the gonorrhoeal virus; this was tested and proved in the usual Hahnemannian manner on many healthy individuals and the symptoms these healthy provers produced were carefully noted down and if a sick person shows a number of these symptoms, *Med.* will cure. Let me recapitulate them: choking cough, larynx feels as if closed up, so that no air could enter, only improved by lying on face, deep hollow cough worse lying down, better lying on stomach, difficult respiration, wants to be fanned, feels cold, yet throws the covers off, also is made worse by warmth, even when icy cold to touch, worse by wet, damp, draught and thunderstorms, worse from daylight to sunset, always brighter in the evenings. The general condition is better near the seashore and worse inland. Has burning feet, wants them uncovered and likes to be fanned. Introspective, self-accusative, remorseful, time moves too slowly, therefore always in a hurry, history of smallpox, vaccination or gonorrhoea, *if you can get it.*

It is no use prescribing on one symptom only, you must have several, in order to get at the right remedy. For example, under the symptoms 'difficult respiration, wants to be fanned' you find seven remedies; so you have to individualize. I had an asthmatic patient some years ago, where I had great difficulty in finding the right medicine. She was round about sixty, had been a hard working cook in her time, but was hardly able to crawl about because of constant attacks of bronchial asthma; she took aspirin — why I never found out — to relieve the attacks, it did not really make any difference though. She had dropsy in her feet and legs up to her knees, albumen in her urine, chest full of many adventitious sounds, moist râles, dry whistling sounds. Not at all a nice case to tackle, her heart sounds were feeble and rapid; her face looked grey and drawn, especially during an attack. I tried various remedies, *Ars.*, *Ipecac.*, *etc.*, with no appreciable effect. Eventually her symptoms cleared and one got the following: difficult respiration, wants air, has always a fan near her, attack is preceded by a great feeling of heat which lasts right through the breathless period; attacks < while lying down. Wants windows and doors wide open. I gave her *Carbo veg.* and was disappointed that there was no change in the condition. In looking over the case again, one saw *Apis* as the indicated remedy: she felt the heat very much, did not like to sit too near the fire, she was fearful and sad, had oedema; even though *Apis* was not mentioned specifically as a remedy for asthma, *Apis* covered the symptoms here, and after *Apis* we saw the first signs of improvement. She was able to be about in quite a short time, the oedema and albuminuria cleared up and the bronchitis and asthma became bearable. She was kept on *Apis* 6 t.d.s. and after a short while she took it only during an attack; during the whole summer which usually was her worst time she improved, then, *Apis.* 12 nightly was taken; when that potency did not act any more, *Apis* 30 was necessary, we worked up gradually to *Apis* 200 and *Apis* 1m. *Apis* altered her condition so much and built up her constitution, that from being a bed-ridden woman, she was able to get about easily, do her own house-work and cooking, her own washing, even as to sheets and blankets.

She still occasionally gets attacks of breathlessness when she hurries, or when the wind is in the east, and is very liable to catch colds and chills, but then she is well over seventy and she does not look it. *Apis* put her on her feet, and you ask her what she thinks of Homoeopathy! What a difference it has made to her life. *Apis* is also an anti-sycotic remedy, even though *Carbo veg.* seemed to be indicated at first, it did not cover all the symptoms, it was not strongly enough sycotic. The sycosis in this case was probably derived from vaccination, as she had been 'done' two or three times.

When the asthma got better, she developed troublesome feet and painful bunions; proving another important axiom of the law of cure. The disease goes from the more important to the lesser organ.

She is now about 75, keeping well, asthmatic attacks are rare. Kept in check now with *Puls.* 6, when necessary. She is emotional, weeps easily and likes sympathy, hence the change in the remedy.

In 1947, three years later, she is still free from asthma: even old people can be cured, provided they keep away from adrenalin and other palliatives.

Silica is another sycotic remedy and one of the greatest cures for asthma, inveterate cases of catarrh of the chest, with asthmatic wheezing, tremulous suffocation, inability to move, brought on by over-heating and over-exertion. A person over-exerts herself, gets hot, and then becomes exposed to a draught. Humid asthma, coarse rattling, and the whole chest seems full of mucus, as if she would suffocate. Usually asthma of old sycotics, or children of such. The complexion is pale, waxy, anaemic, with great prostration and thirst. (Kent.) Comes on after suppressed gonorrhoea — from suppressed perspiration and foot-sweat — which is usually very foetid — feels cold, is sensitive to draughts and thunderstorms — head sweats. If there is a patient with all or most of these symptoms, you will find *Silica* will quickly eradicate the trouble, and by eradication I mean, the asthma attacks will get less and less and eventually disappear.

I mentioned the *Kali* salts earlier on as being sycotic remedies, suitable for this complaint.

There is *Kali Arsenicosum*: the old familiar Fowler's solution of our student days, very little used in Homoeopathy, but *when indicated*, it works like a charm.

Remedies, in my mind, are frequently associated with people, and this one always recalls a nurse of the old hospital days who was trained in the days of the paying lady probationers. She was spartan, practical, competent and very, very stern, managed her house-committee with a rod of iron, they dared not say anything to her, but just bow to the inevitable and pay the bills for the things she considered necessary for the small hospital of which she was in charge.

Her one disability was her tendency to asthma and bronchitis; she felt the cold terribly, suffered from lack of vital heat, felt draughts, her rooms were like a hot-house, and oh! the clothes she wore, layers and layers of thick flannel (even in summer), she was comparatively slim when she had shed the two or three petticoats and vests and other impedimenta. She panted of course on ascending stairs and during exertion, her lungs were full of moist catarrhal sounds; her bronchitis was better in the warmth and warm drinks relieved, specially Ovaltine. Her condition was always worse between 2-3 a.m., that hour was purgatory to her and she dreaded it; specially every third day she would be suffering the tortures of the damned. Very restless during the attacks. Well, *Kali ars.* 6 t.d.s., cured the bronchial asthma in a few days and kept her free for months, and aborted the trouble several times. Eventually she had to retire and at well over eighty went to live in the backwaters of Wales where she succumbed two or three years later during an attack of bronchial asthma under the care of a local doctor.

The other *Kali* salt useful for asthma is *Kali carb.* I have already mentioned it previously; see the case of the boy who attended the dispensary for months and did not get any relief until by chance he let on that his attacks were worse between 3 and 5 a.m.

Why is it, can anybody tell me, that some asthma cases are like alarm clocks set for a certain time, always awakened at the same time? There is no pathological reason for it that I can see and yet a *Kali ars.* patient wakens regularly at 2 a.m. and is worse between 2-3 a.m.; a *Kali carb.* patient is worse between 2 or 3-4 or 5 a.m., e.g. he starts at 2 a.m. and goes on to 5 a.m. A *Nat. sulph.* patient does not get roused until 4 a.m. and eases up after 5 a.m.

On the other hand *Ars.* starts about midnight and his worst spell is between 12 and 2 a.m. If you get periodicity and the special time signals, pay attention to it and give the remedy according to these indications and the trouble will improve rapidly. Of course, Summer Time might throw you out in your calculations, so make allowances for it!

Kali carb. has one of the most violent coughs which comes on with great choking and suffocation between the hours mentioned. Lying down is impossible, he must sit up, sit forward with head on table or knees, he cannot bear any draughts, feels the cold very much and is worse in cold, foggy weather and is usually a pale sickly and anaemic person and complains of stitching wandering pains in the chest, which come on irrespective of motion, different from *Bryonia*, which has stitching pains, worse motion, worse coughing, and the chest is cold. Frequently you may notice also a baggy swelling between the eyelids and eyebrows when *Kali carb.* is needed.

Talking of periodicity and time aggravations in medicines, I must just refer to *Aralia*, the American spikenard. As far as I know, this has not been proved to be a sycotic remedy, but if a patient has the following symptoms, it will wipe them out at once, as has been shown again and again. The patient goes to sleep and is awakened at 11 p.m. or just before midnight, immediately on lying down or more commonly after a short sleep, by a violent cough caused by a tickling in the throat with constriction of chest, has to sit up and cough violently or he would choke. All obstruction seems to be in the inspiratory effort. The sputum is warm and saltish.

The prover, a doctor himself, developed a violent attack of asthma with these afore-mentioned symptoms and ever since *Aralia* has proved effective when these symptoms are present in a sick person.

Sambucus nigra, the elder bush, is another remedy which produces and therefore cures spasmodic respiratory troubles of the larynx and chest with a definite time periodicity. The child, it is mainly a children's remedy, awakens suddenly at 3 a.m., it sleeps into the attack like *Lachesis* and *Aralia* — only it comes on later than *Aralia* — is nearly suffocated, face livid and blue, it has to sit up in bed, gasping for breath, finally it gets its breath, then goes to sleep again, to be awakened again with another attack. Another peculiarity of *Sambucus* is: profuse sweat when awake and dry heat during sleep. Snuffles in the nose are very often present.

Lachesis is another remedy with slightly sycotic tendencies — which has similar aggravations, the asthmatic attacks may occur during sleep and never waken the person (like *Sulph.*), they may also come on when falling asleep and on first waking up in the morning.

The patient, usually a woman during the climacteric, who requires *Lachesis* for her asthma would show the strong *Lachesis* characteristics. That is, she would suffer from the heat, her asthma would come on from any constriction round the throat or even if the throat was touched, or if her mouth or nose were covered, say she fell asleep and burrowed with her head under the bed-clothes, she would have an attack, which might not even wake her, but would disturb and waken her husband. It would come on after violently moving her arms and a long gossip with her neighbours over the teacups would precipitate an attack. Suffering with great heat she must have windows and doors open, just the same as a *Pulsatilla* or *Apis* or *Sulphur* patient, only the concomitant symptoms would be different. You could spot a *Lachesis* patient by her purplish or bluish complexion, a woman who would look at you with very suspicious eyes, her husband might give the fact away too that she was extremely jealous, and you would soon notice that in spite of her breathlessness, she was loquacious and talkative. It is more frequently indicated in cardiac asthma, rather than in bronchial asthma.

You see how carefully one has to watch each patient, how one has to get all the information one can from the husband or the wife or a relative who is in close touch with the sufferer, or a nurse who is attending, as well as getting all the subjective sensations and symptoms from the patient.

Dr. Roberts in one of his books mentions a case of chronic asthma, who was complaining of the characteristic wheezing, suffocative sensation and such-like symptoms. 'How can we prescribe on these symptoms?' he says. These are common symptoms, common to the complaint; there are nearly 150 remedies mentioned in Kent for asthma. You have to find out the distinctive symptoms, such individual symptoms which distinguish the particular patient from any other case. This patient's cough was worse at night, and better after expectoration; his hands and feet were cold.

This immediately limited the number of remedies which had to be considered to about ten remedies. Then he added that the cough was worse from drinking water, which reduced the number of remedies to four: and lastly he mentioned the most enlightening symptom yet related. It seemed as if a choking sensation was rising up from his stomach into his throat and suffocating him and which brought on the attack. There are but two remedies to be thought of with this symptom, namely *Sepia* and *Mancinella* (most). The provings of *Mancinella* brought out this symptom phrased by the provers exactly as this patient described it. By comparing these two remedies and looking them up in the Materia Medica, it was found that *Mancinella* was the remedy. That is how a master works; and the symptom which helped to find the right remedy was what is called a strange, rare, and peculiar symptom: strange and rare as regards the particular complaint, and peculiar to the individual.

Now follows the details of working out a remedy on symptoms given with the help of a homoeopathic repertory:

(1) Cough at nights and expectoration ameliorates. Bell.; Calc.; Carbo. an.; Caust.; Hep.; *Ipecac.*; Kali nit.; Kreos.; Lach.; Manc.; Mez.; *Sep.*

(2) Coldness of hands and feet: Bell.; Calc.; Carb. an.; Caust.; Hep.; *Ipecac.*; Lach.; Manc.; Mez.; *Sep.*

(3) Cough on drinking water: Calc.; Hep.; *Lach.*; *Manc.*

(4) Choking sensation rising up from stomach into throat, and suffocating him, which brings on the attack:

MANC.; Sep. (extracted from a Homoeopathic repertory), and so *Mancinella* was the remedy which proved
effective.

Lucky is the physician who finds such a patient, who is
sufficiently intelligent and observant to relate his sufferings
in such a way that the remedy which cures can be found.
Sometimes it requires much patience on the doctor's part and
much delving into the past history and much questioning and
long observation before all the important factors can be
elucidated.

One of the easiest cases for finding the correct remedy was
the case already referred to of the pilot – a captain on the
west coast – and a story well worth repeating, who always
had asthma ashore; as long as he was out at sea, he was
perfectly all right, but he did not like the land, it would
always stir up his asthma. He was a big, stout man, weighing
well over 18 stones, very fair and blue eyed – a typical sailor.
Well, his remedy was *Bromine* and *Bromine* 6 t.d.s., for a
short period of time made a vast difference to him. A
Bromine patient is very like a *Pulsatilla* patient, and *Bromine*
steps in where *Pulsatilla* fails. *Bromine* constricts the larynx,
the glottis closes spasmodically. There is a feeling of coldness
in the larynx, the air breathed feels cold, just as if it were
blown off from a glacier. Another peculiar sensation the
Bromine patient has is: as if the air passages were full of
smoke. Any kind of dust makes it worse; that is why a sailor
is free at sea, but the dust ashore starts up his trouble again.
Bromine is frequently indicated in the asthma of children; a
fat, fair, blue-eyed child, who on board ship – on a
cruise – is free from asthma, but develops it again on land.
One seems to recall the remarks of a certain journalist who in
his chatty letters owns up to frequent attacks of bronchitis
and asthma, and who apparently is always free on the
transatlantic crossings. Some Homoeopathy seems indicated!
Unfortunately Lord C. the journalist mentioned died from
asthma, shortly after this was written.

We have seen that sycosis is a frequent cause of chronic
asthma, and mentioned several sycotic remedies which act

well in its treatment, but there are other constitutional defects which produce asthma.

There is the tubercular constitution which may be in the background; when asthma does not respond to the apparently indicated remedy, then it is very wise to interpolate some *Tuberculinum* in a high potency at infrequent intervals. There may be no evidence of a pathological character, no *Bacillus Tub.* will be found in the sputum; yet there are definite homoeopathic indications why *Tub.* should be given. These people are always tired, born tired, the tired Tims of this world; debilitated, anaemic, with fair silken, often curly hair, transparent skin, long eyelashes, blue eyes and blue sclerotics with fine hair growing along the spine. Always taking cold with each breath of fresh air, even though there is a craving for fresh air, a love for being out in the cold wind and storm. It was Shelley, I think, who loved driving out in a storm and who unfortunately died in the early twenties of rapid consumption.

One should always ask, when taking a patient's history, whether there has been T.B. in the family. Sometimes you get the required information by asking 'is there any chest trouble in your family?' followed up by 'what is it?' If you find out that some member or members of the family succumbed to the white plague, then you have a short cut to your remedy, specially if you find some other symptoms such as I mentioned previously: love of being out in storms, taking colds easily from draughts; the pretty doll-like, delicate appearance of the patient — usually they are not satisfied with staying at home, they love change, like to travel and roam, to run away from school or from their homes. Then in such cases, you cannot go far wrong, the asthma will clear up and the whole constitution will alter, the child or young adult will become robust and suddenly take a new lease of life and will cease to be an anxiety to the family.

Drosera is another tubercular remedy; but there are more spasms, more paroxysms of cough in this medicine. The asthmatic breathing comes on from spasms in the larynx, from talking, with a deep sounding, hoarse cough; asthma which remains after whooping-cough or measles; worse lying down after midnight and towards early morning, a 2 a.m. cough; with tickling in the larynx and stitching in the chest, must press on the chest with the hands for relief. The cough is so violent that the patient almost goes into convulsions.

In these violent paroxysms of cough, always remember *Drosera*, specially if there is a T.B. history — and give it with great caution! *Drosera* is a deep-acting and slow-acting medicine, and should not be repeated rashly. If *Drosera* is indicated, give one dose and wait. You get quick results if it is given correctly. The patient puts on weight by leaps and bounds, and the cough disappears like magic. If there is no alteration in the cough and the patient does not put on weight rapidly, you will have to alter your prescription — give one of the *Kali* salts (worse early morning, worse 3 a.m.).

There may be a syphilitic taint in the family; you will not get an acknowledgment of this stigma; it is indeed a secret disease, secret except to the eye which sees and the mind with knowledge and training. For though secret, it cannot be hidden, it comes out duly for several generations — the sins of the fathers show for three or four generations. The syphilitic patient is always worse at night, so with a severe night cough — when the patient dreads the night — keep a syphilitic remedy in mind, it will alter the case; asthma in warm, damp weather, during the night — an unusual symptom except in the syphilitic. I had a patient once — a girl who always had asthma during a thunderstorm at night, and *Syph.* proved to be the remedy. Dyspnoea worse nights, worse 1-4 a.m., perfectly placid during the day, but the moment the night comes on, cough and suffocation and breathlessness with pain behind sternum, a feeling as if the chest were gradually drawn towards the dorsal vertebrae (the spine).

You see, each constitution has its own peculiar symptoms, which stamps it and thus points the way to a cure. Thus *Drosera* or *Tuberculinum* in a tubercular case, *Medorrhinum* in a sycotic family and *Syphilinum* in a syphilitic family: each show different signs and symptoms, and if properly given, would eradicate the particular taint. Once the constitutional taint is removed, the symptoms will alter and the patient will recover, provided there is not a combination of taints. In some unfortunate families, you will find a mixture of syphilis and sycosis and tuberculosis, truly a hell's broth — the real complication of diseases, and then it means a slow unravelling of the case, at one time one taint is uppermost and that particular taint will have to be antidoted, and then another disease stigma comes up, and this will have to be treated and removed by the right remedy. But if the victim has faith and patience, he or she can be made, if not whole — at any rate much stronger. Two or three complete generations would have to be treated *secundum artem* — according to Homoeopathy, in order to eradicate all the mixtures of constitutional stigmatization. We are all victims of our forefathers' failings and shortcomings and we cannot be blamed for it. Our responsibility to the succeeding generation is not to add our quota, not to make it worse, but to diminish it, if possible, by simple, healthy living, and by refraining from vicious acts and thoughts.

But to go back to asthma:

Rumex crispus, the yellow dock, which is a common British weed, once stood me in good stead with a case of asthma in a nurse. Nurses are proverbially known to be great critics of a doctor's treatment, and I converted this nurse to Homoeopathy through the rapid cure of her asthma by *Rumex*. She was out visiting some cases on a raw and cold December morning, when she was suddenly seized in the street with inability to breathe deeply and paroxysms of cough which took her breath away. She struggled into a chemist's shop near by and was given some ephedrine which temporarily relieved the spasm somewhat. She felt so ill however that she went home to bed. I saw her three days later and noticed her bad colour and her breathlessness; she had exhausting paroxysms of cough in spite of the ephedrine which made her feel much worse now and gave her indigestion and discomfort after food.

I persuaded her to give up the ephedrine and try the little

sugar pills instead. The cough always began with tickling behind the top of the sternum (throat pit). She could not bear the pressure of her collar round the throat.

Any change of temperature going from warm room to the cold air outside or vice versa brought on violent attacks of coughing. She also had a feeling of rawness under the clavicles and even though the cough was violent, shaking the chest and head, the expectoration was scanty and difficult to raise.

She was very distressed and upset about it all, for the Christmas recess was just due the next day and she wanted to go to her people in Cardiff. I was extremely doubtful whether she would be fit to travel; but she was adamant about it. She was given *Rumex* 30, 3-hourly, and I reckoned that even if she got as far as Cardiff, she would not be well enough to return under a fortnight. In fact I was very anxious about her and afraid that the cold raw weather might give her pneumonia on top of her asthma; five days later, after the holiday, I saw her again – asthma gone, chest clear! She arrived at Cardiff in the evening very exhausted and done up, but a hot meal, a night's sleep and the pills made her feel a new creature, so that she was able to enjoy the yearly festivities. And the asthma did not come back either after her return to London, so the cessation of the attack was *not* due to the change of habitat, but due to the action of the medicine.

And note in this case too, she had several doses of ephedrine which sometimes is helpful in cutting short acute attacks of asthma, but with her it seemed to add to the discomfort by giving her dyspepsia. It was very risky going on a long journey during an attack of bronchial asthma, but the indicated remedy here, *Rumex* – cured rapidly. *Rumex* 10*m* on her return finished off the cure.

Another remedy has often helped me in old people, namely *Senega*. This is a common ingredient as an adjuvant to the allopathic cough mixture in half oz. doses. We give it in very minute doses and it works better still.

The cough is like a *Rumex* cough, it comes on, on first

going into the cold air and is a dry, violent cough, with difficult expectoration. There was a very old lady, some twenty years ago, well over 80, quite active and brisk except for these frequent attacks of asthma, and she got easily and safely through two or three attacks every winter for about five years with *Senega*. I gave it her in the 15th potency, the only one I had got, at 3-hourly intervals. Her chest used to be full of loud coarse râles, the mucus was so tough and ropy she could not raise it, she was always gagging and coughing, the throat was so dry and yet in less than a week we had conquered the asthma and the phlegm came up easily and the cough had almost disappeared. The dear old lady was always so grateful, one of the world's smilers, always a cheery word for everyone, it did one good to be with her. She used to say: 'I am always so breathless, I can only sit propped up in bed, and I rattle and rattle and wheeze, and I feel my chest is like a water-bag so full and I can't raise the phlegm, and then after one dose of medicine which is almost tasteless, I feel so different, I can lie down better, I can sleep and the weight goes and the breathlessness goes: such a blessed relief! — and with the other doctors, I had to go on taking their stuff all the winter. I was in bed for weeks and never left the room for months. I can hardly believe it is possible that something which tastes like water can make such a difference.'

Yes, I must be allowed to express my gratitude to Dr. Nash — for it was due to his tip which I read in one of his books — rattling chest, especially valuable in old people — which enabled me to cure this old lady and many other old people since; one does not always meet with gratitude, or even recognition on getting a patient well quickly.

This was a Civil Servant, I have in mind — a history of asthma for years — had her turbinated bones sliced off and curetted so that her nose did not fulfil its action of being a filter any more. The right nostril was full of adhesions after two or three operations; her antrum had been drained, and yet the attacks became rather worse than better. There was great weakness in the chest, great dyspnoea, extreme cyanosis and blueness of the face and lips, the wings of the nostrils moved rapidly all the time; a short, dry hacking cough, frequently finishing off with a belch or even sickness, her chest felt so weak and full of burning stitching pains; frightful oppression and suffocation of the chest, so great that the only relief she got was by hanging the legs down; this caused such inconvenience that she would not stay in bed, but preferred to sit up in a chair. Fretful and irritable, nothing could please her, and when well, I know, she was always in a hurry and a flurry; could not work fast enough. *Sulphuric acid* was her remedy, and it just seemed to make a new woman of her. The terrible asthma disappeared and the nurse who looked after her had never seen a severe case of bronchial asthma clear up so quickly! She was free for weeks and months, and the next attack she had, she was so angry at having another one, she went back to the Adrenalin and the Ephedrine, and she has never been free from asthma since; acute violent explosions every few days and chronic breathlessness all the time. Homoeopathy is no good, she says, even though she was told it might come back and would require treatment for months. She prefers to suffer and take Ephedrine!

Yes, asthma patients are awkward bodies to deal with, more so if they have been well soaked through and through with allopathic medication. They are extremely nervous people anyhow, or they would not have asthma and this, combined with the antispasmodic, analgesic, pain-killing drugs they swallow makes them hateful. Years of treatment with such strong poisons as Adrenalin, Ephedrine, Cocaine and Morphia compounds — though the two latter are rarely met with now, since the Poison Drug Acts have been passed — sours their outlook, alters their temperament and turns them into suspicious, jealous, disagreeable, backbiting people, people it is wiser not to offend and to steer clear of.

I knew a nasal surgeon, years ago, before the 1st World War, whose character was sadly altered by constant inhalations and sprays of Cocaine and Adrenalin. He never trusted anybody, so suspicious that he would not believe a word anybody said to him, a liar himself; sly, always creeping round the hospital, spying out trouble, making mischief where he could — a most unpleasant gentleman. *Requiescat in pace.* Everybody in that hospital was relieved when he passed on; and yet somebody told me he used to be a very nice man when he was younger. It gave me a horror of asthmatics and so-called cures for asthma. I met a woman a year or two later, a chronic asthmatic sufferer for fifty years, with exactly the same creeping walk and the bent figure and the sly expression and the mischief-making tendency — even though she was a professed nun in an enclosed order, and I recognised the effects of the poisonous, character-undermining drugs she had taken for half a lifetime. Yes, the cures are often worse than the disease!

Never start an asthma patient on the downward path of the various asthma cures, which they have to go on taking in ever increasing doses, yet this is called a cure! There is no logic in such a statement, but then logic is not considered necessary these days.

Recently I met a woman doctor working in a well-known children's hospital who was lamenting the fact that present-day medication made very little impression on the small asthma patients. Endless tests were made for protein sensitization, cat's hair, horse hair, hen's feathers, various articles of food were tested for reaction. The lists of tests were an ever-lengthening one, and the effects on the disease were nil! You are just as wise after having made all these tests as you were before, and the patient is left battling with his disease. Kapok pillows are prescribed, because feathers are said to invite attacks; elaborate breathing exercises have been worked out, which entail attendance at the massage department several times a week for months. Exercises improve the deformed chest wall, I admit and tone up the general metabolism, but do not cure the asthma, not as thoroughly and effectively as the indicated remedy, the simillimum. I have tried for years by means of exercises and artificial sunlight alone to overcome asthma, and never, never did I get good results until I used Homoeopathy.

Now for another case history, this time in a woman of 54, first seen in September, 1937, who had asthma for years, just as her father had, which proved there was an unstable nervous system in the family. Six years ago she had an operation for gallstones and partial excision of gall bladder; in spite of which she still gets violent attacks of indigestion and gallstone colic, the last one was two weeks ago; very constipated, bowels do not move without an aperient. Has used aluminium saucepans for years.

Asthma comes on with flatulence. Milk gives her indigestion, asthma is worse at the seaside, indeed it started at the seaside. Cannot take vegetables, very fond of sweets which disagree. Very thin woman, excitable, artistic, loves music, used to be a singer and, in spite of breathing exercises, asthma got worse and worse, in the end she had to give up singing.

On these symptoms, *Magnesium mur.*, one dose was given, and *Colocynth* 30 was to be dissolved in half a tumblerful of water and taken half-hourly for the acute attacks of pain and vomiting for which she used to get Morphia injections from her panel doctor.

Of course she was dieted as well: brown bread, bran, bran porridge, bran scones and cakes were ordered; fruit and tomatoes were to be taken daily, oranges were forbidden and aluminium saucepans were banned; junket, whey, Marmite, white of eggs and glucose were strongly recommended.

Ten days later, constipation much improved; she has not taken any other medicines. *Colocynth* relieves attacks of pain; feels cold very much even in hot weather; tongue which used to be thickly furred is much cleaner. Examined her spine and adjusted the 6th and 7th cervical and the 8th dorsal vertebrae. Had urticaria as a child in the spring, which is another sign of allergy. — Continue *Colocynth* 30 when neccssary.

12.10.37. A month later. Woke up with asthma at 4 a.m. Worse damp weather, asthma worse after flatulence, usually spends the winter indoors, as the wet and the cold give her asthma. Worse milk, worse green vegetables; always has asthma when she goes to Brighton. *Natrum sulph.* 30 (one dose) and *Colocynth* as before for acute indigestion.

18.11.37. Acute attack of influenza with bronchial symptoms; Temperature 102. Respiration 40. Pulse 120. *Bryonia* 30, half-hourly. District nurse came in; temperature down in 36 hours, after *Bryonia* was sent; ill for two days before letting me know. *Kali phos.* 200, three doses in 24 hours, prescribed for debility after influenza. No asthma with or after influenza, quite unlike previous feverish chills she has had.

29.12.37. Attack of lumbago, similar to the one she had after her operation six years ago (return of old symptoms). Had chicken at Christmas and a glass of Sauterne and enjoyed it; wine used to disagree. Much better, has been going out much more, which she has not been able to do for years.

Colocynth acts like a charm when she has indigestion and flatulence. No asthma since early in October. Had feverish attack just before Christmas, which two doses of *Bryonia* aborted. The breath sounds which in September sounded like an orchestra, are quite normal. No breathlessness now. 1. *Mag. mur.* 30 (one dose). 2. *Colocynth* 30, p.r.n. (as need).

25.1.38. Slight flatulence and pain after working about and lifting things, able to do her own house work now; rather overdoes it. Always has had asthma every November for years; one doctor advised her to go to Egypt every year for the winter!

No trouble with asthma this November. Looks fat and well; has put on weight. *Colocynth* 30, p.r.n.

4.4.38. Attack of asthma after spring cleaning; looked so well, hardly recognised her. Repeat *Mag. mur.* 30 (one dose).

18.5.38. Attack of asthma again. *Mag. mur.* 30, three doses on three consecutive nights.

6.10.38. No asthma for five months. Chest much better, indigestion troublesome after milk; white motions, liver still troublesome, fat disagrees; very nervous of noise. *Natrum carb.* 30 (one dose).

September 29th, 1939. Just after the start of the war which upset her emotionally. Looks so well and plump. I had difficulty in recognising her. Pain side of chest going through to back; feeling of suffocation with perspiration; flatulence. *Carbo veg.* 6 t.d.s.

5.7.40. Very well until last week: some cough again. *Carbo veg.* 6, night and morning.

22.7.40. Got drenched in thunderstorm: worse wet weather, cough and indigestion; pain at side in liver region. *Nat. sulph.* 30 (one dose) and *Colocynth* 30, p.r.n.

26.8.40. Asthma again, digestion poor, has been working very hard; return of old symptoms similar to those she had when she first came to me. *Mag. mur.* 30, three doses in 24 hours.

I heard recently, that she has been very well since; no asthma and no indigestion; is working hard.

It is not easy to cure a woman suffering from gallstone colic and asthma of many years standing with ordinary medical treatment. Her life was a misery to her, and how quickly she responded to the remedies selected for her. Individualize each case, whatever the diagnosis may be, and if the patient is willing to assist you by giving a correct account of her sufferings, Homoeopathy can be of the greatest use, and can frequently turn a broken vessel into a sound one.

Advertisements tell you: 'Take such and such a cure, it will give you instant relief.' Yes, but you have to go on taking the cure; it does not stop it permanently, while Homoeopathy if given time will prevent recurrence. The majority among the medical and nursing professions deny this; they have never seen a cure, therefore a cure is impossible, unfortunately they make it difficult for those who wish to give Homoeopathy a chance. The parents of a child suffering from asthma on looking round for a real cure were told of a doctor who was 'simply marvellous with asthma, you know'. His own wife was a chronic asthmatic and continued having asthma; he was never able to stop the attacks. A trained nurse, matron at the school where this boy was a pupil, refused to give him his pills, as she had a mother who had asthma all her life and she knew exactly what to do; the mother lived and died an asthmatic, consequently the daughter knew all about it; but she did not know the most important thing: that Homoeopathy can cure asthma so completely that the attacks stop, provided the patient and relatives co-operate. Give up taking the various 'cures' which only relieve the immediate attack and give nature, that is the vital force of the individual in question, the chance to cure from within so that in time the patient may go to sleep in a horse-box if he likes and never have an attack, even though he may have been sensitive to horse hair according to the tests. He may have as many cats as he likes near him and again need not fear an attack, he will become immune to cat's hair. Is this not much more satisfactory than being continually afraid of certain things and worth taking trouble over in order to bring it about?

Amidst all this welter of diagnostic refinements, have we not forgotten that the principal object of medicine is or should be the real cure of the sick person? A cure does not mean a suppression of the symptoms, so that in a short time the disease bobs up again under a different name. A cure means making the individual so well that he forgets that he is ill and enjoys life and dies, not from a disease but from old age, without having been a burden to his relatives and friends.

CHAPTER FIVE

COLDS AND CHILLS

Many thousand working hours are lost every year through colds and feverish chills, and workers are laid aside unnecessarily and insurance companies have to pay out large sums of money. There is no certain fool-proof method for preventing colds, indeed it is just that a cold has got to go through its different stages without help or hindrance — even the doctors themselves are not immune to it — unless you are skilled in Homoeopathy.

I am often asked what cure Homoeopathy has for colds and feverish chills. Well, there is no specific cure; it depends on so many different factors. As always, study the symptoms your patient presents and according to what you find, you will be able to, or ought to be able to, find the correct remedy to cure a cold.

Nowadays nearly everybody tells you glibly they caught their cold from somebody else; they cannot remember the exact details of the start of the cold which is so important for finding the remedy which will deal with it rapidly. You should remember what the weather was like before you fell a victim to the chill. Was it a windy day, or was it rainy, did you get your feet wet, were you soaked right through; was it a cold damp day, or was it a dry cold wind; did a draught strike your head or your feet or your abdomen? Did the chill come on the same day of the exposure or did it come on gradually and take several days to develop? Some people are more sensitive to dry cold weather, some feel the wet more; others are affected by the cold and the wet, and some by warm, wet spells. Some get chills in warm, wet winters; others are laid low, when the wind is dry and blows from the north. One and all are covered by different medicines, and it means hard work for a doctor to find out all the details and find the right remedy. You are a first-class homoeopath if you can cure a cold rapidly; it is none too easy. I fail very often, I must confess, a cold often beats me; it is really largely the patient's fault, they forget how it started, they take their own patent cures first, and by the time the doctor sees the patient, the cold is well on the way. Still Homoeopathy can be very helpful. There was a middle-aged lady, I remember, who was always catching colds which went down to her chest rapidly. She had her favourite cough medicines which she always took, without much effect it is true. In the spring of 1941, which was very cold and changeable, she got a violent chill, was shivery and had to sit over the fire wrapped up even with a shawl over her head. She would not give in, but had to go to bed eventually. After four or five days in bed she crawled back to work, looking miserable, coughing, and with a severe running cold. She could not shake it off, it got worse and for six weeks she was fighting this cold and cough. In the end a surgeon, whom she consulted about something else and who noticed her plight, sent her to me. I found she suffered from a terrible tickle behind the top of the sternum, in the throat part, the trachea was raw inside and sore to pressure; exhausting paroxyms of coughing with scanty expectoration which was difficult to raise. The coughing and sneezing was worse before midnight; regularly about 11 p.m. she had a terrible spell of it. She looked ghastly and felt ghastly, not fit to be out of bed. I prescribed *Rumex* 30 for her in four-hourly doses and saw her two days later. She was smiling happily and looked much better. All the symptoms had improved. 'Could she have some more of those wonderful powders?' She was given *Rumex* 30, three times daily and went off on a week's holiday which she spent travelling up and down the Thames in the little river steamers; fortunately it was beautifully fine and warm. Result: complete cure and she came back to work looking years younger, and feeling full of energy. A few days' treatment sufficed after she had been ill for six whole weeks!

Yes, *Rumex* does well for these colds which are sensitive to cold air, sensitive to changes in the weather; there is very little feverish reaction, even though there may be a violent coryza which becomes localized eventually in the larynx and trachea with pains behind clavicle and sternum; cough starts with a tickle in the throat, in the notch between the clavicles, and shakes the head and chest and is always at its worst at night about 11 p.m. You may get these symptoms in bronchitis, in influenza, in asthma, and tubercular pthisical cases. The name of the disease does not matter so much. If you get such a cough you can alleviate and cure it rapidly with *Rumex*.

Now for a totally different kind of chill. I know a little girl, who was born with a delicate chest, and has been frequently laid aside with bronchitis and asthma right from infancy. Several times she was ill for weeks and only just escaped death. Then the mother was advised to try Homoeopathy and found the attacks were less frequent and did not last so long. The homoeopath she was under, drew up a strict diet sheet, took her off many articles of food and really set her on the road to health. When he retired, the girlie was transferred to my care. The asthma was on the wane, only very short mild attacks now, but she did manage to get severe bronchial chills every October and February without fail. Under homoeopathic treatment she cleared up invariably in 48 hours or less; but last year she was sent to the country for safety's sake, armed with some homoeopathic medicines and full instructions as to diet, etc. The usual feverish chill turned up punctually as clockwork in October, the dear maiden aunts she stayed with would have nothing to do with Homoeopathy, but being themselves afflicted with 'doctoritis' sent for the local general practitioner, who put the child on a milk diet, even though he was told it did not agree with her, and on the usual fashionable dope, one of the Sulphonamide preparations. Result was as expected, severe bronchitis, a good old asthma attack and a high temperature ranging between 103-104 degrees. This went on for six days, the child was vomiting up everything she took and plaintively remarked she preferred the food, by which she meant the fruit juices, she usually had when she was ill. Her mother got very anxious and hurried to her bedside and bearded the doctor man in his den, as he acknowledged that this case beat him, the mother offered to take the child now and treat her with the medicine which I had sent down by her on the symptoms given, namely *Phos.*: vomiting of everything, even water; great thirst for cold water which was vomited; high temperature, intense heat, red face, tightness of the chest, hard dry hacking cough; lying on the back with head thrown back. *Phos.* 30 diluted in water, was given in half-hourly doses and then hourly doses. The milk was stopped and the child was given orange juice and diluted lemon juice and raisin drink, which is raisins simmered in water for quarter of an hour, strained through a sieve and lemon juice added according to taste — my usual drink for 'chests' which I find most soothing in all bronchial complaints. The vomiting stopped at once, the temperature came down as well and 48 hours later the child was well. The doctor could not understand it at all; and would you believe it, he never had the curiosity to find out how it was done!

In October, 1941, she had a similiar seizure after a chill, which took about 24 hours to develop. Wheezing chest, coughing, and cold immediately which went down from the nose into the chest; vomiting all her food, even water, very little thirst, tongue was clean in spite of the vomiting. The child looked pale, drawn and ill, coarse rattling of the chest, nausea and gagging with the cough. I gave her *Ipecacuanha* 30, hourly doses, and put her on fruit juices — apple juice as nothing else was available. The temperature was 100 degrees in the morning. After vomiting for 12 hours before she had the medicine, she stopped at once after the first dose. In 24 hours the temperature was 99 degrees and 48 hours later she was normal, the breathing was quiet and peaceful, she had slept well, even the first night after the *Ipecacuanha*.

On the Friday morning, two days after she had taken to bed, she was well, was put back on a fish and bread and butter diet, which she greatly enjoyed; and all was well. How different from the treatment the previous year under the orthodox régime!

Chills can be aborted. Here in London I find *Arsenic* is the

usual remedy required to stop a chill in the early stages —
sneezing from every change in the weather, always chilly,
suffering from draughts, worse in cold damp weather. The
cold begins in the nose and goes down to the throat, the
discharge from the nose is thin and watery, there is frontal
headache and the patient is restless, anxious and somewhat
distressed and thirsty for small sips of warm water. Burning
of the throat with redness of the mucous membrane.

I have seen dozens of people with such symptoms and a
few doses of *Ars.* 6 or 30 removes the chill in a few hours.

I once saw a dental surgeon at 10 a.m. who complained of
a feverish chill, temperature 100. *Ars.* 30 half-hourly. By 2
o'clock she was hard at it doing a busy gas session, extracting
the teeth, under anaesthetic, of over 30 children. Was rung up
by father in the late afternoon who having heard she was
having 'flu, wanted to commiserate. My dentist had forgotten
all about it, said she felt extremely flourishing and well; never
turned a hair afterwards. The sceptic would say, 'she just
worked it off, it was a lucky fluke'. Only it happens so many
times, that that theory does not work; it is not coincidence,
but hard fact.

I myself do not develop *Arsenic* chills, my colds are
generally aborted, or cured rapidly, by either *Nux vom.* or
Pulsatilla.

The *Nux vom.* chill, coryza or influenza, according to the
severity of the symptoms, comes on after exposure to a dry,
cold wind. The coryza is worse in the evening, worse in the
house, so troublesome in a warm bed that the discharge runs
all over the pillow, better for cool air. With a feverish chill
Nux vom. will cure, when the chilly feeling, beginning in the
extremities or back, runs all over the body, and the patient
must remain covered up; as soon as he moves and raises the
bed-clothes he is cold and shivery. Then he gets hot and
perspires, but still he must remain covered up throughout all
these stages.

The *Nux vom.* patient is irritable, short and snappy and
growling; almost impossible to live with peacefully while he is
ill.

The *Pulsatilla* chill or coryza is somewhat different, sneezing and stuffiness of the nose, with pains in the face and through the nose, worse in a warm room, better when moving about in the open air; cheeks feel hot; the cold starts after getting soaked through, or at any rate after getting feet wet. There is rapid loss of smell and loss of taste; the discharge, at first copious and watery, soon becomes thick, greenish-yellow and bland. The chilly feeling starts in the back, running up and down back, as if cold water was poured down the back.

I remember a chill coming on as I described just now. I took one dose of *Puls.* 10*m* in the evening and in less than an hour I felt well and all trace of a cold had completely disappeared by the morning. Another time I was away from home and only had *Puls.* 6 handy. I had to take several doses and I took over 24 hours to get well. But then I knew my constitution, I know I can take high potencies and react well to them. Also you have to strike the absolute simillimum, the most like. drug in a high potency or you will do no good, or even may do harm. If you are not sure of your remedy, a low potency will do more good, even if it is not the most exact drug wanted, and do less harm than a high potency given wrongly.

Some homoeopaths swear by *Allium cepa* for a cold. It should do well after exposure to cold, damp winds. You get rawness in the nose, copious streaming flow of water from the eyes which is always bland and an excoriating, burning, copious watery discharge from the nose which burns and excoriates the lips. The rawness of the throat quickly extends into the chest. There is tearing in the larynx as if it was torn with a hook, and he has to hold and grasp the larynx during a fit of coughing. Usually the trouble begins on the left side: the left eye and left nostril are affected first and then it spreads over to the other side. The tickling in the larynx, the cough from inhaling cold air and the tearing pain in the larynx is worse in the warm room and worse in the evening.

If you get a combination of symptoms like this, *Allium cepa* will cure rapidly.

A.B. Girl, 18 years. Chill: frontal headache, backache, legs feel heavy and tired; 'faint and queer', Temperature 100°. Pulse 98. Weather changeable, had been snowing and raining alternately for several days previous. Seen in bed next day. Temperature 100°. Pulse 96.

Patient heavy and dazed, no desire to move; cough, rawness behind sternum; nausea; anorexia, feverish, dry heat, no perspiration; no thirst; sleepless all night. Main complaint was chilliness in bed, *feeling of cold water running down spine. Puls.* 1*m*, one dose given.

The next day patient was sitting up in bed reading the newspaper, had a good night. Temperature 99°. Pains in legs and backache gone. Asked whether she still felt the cold water flowing down her back, she replied: 'Oh no, I have not noticed that since yesterday afternoon.' Patient was up and about in three days. Cough gave her no more trouble, she was back at her work a week later, while her sister, who gave the cold to A.B. still visited her allopathic doctor for 'another bottle of medicine' for her cough a fortnight after.

Baby, 2 years old. Croupy cough for several days after being exposed to a cold wind. Much choking, rattling in chest, always worse at night. Warm baby, always throws off its covers. *Calc. sulph.* 10*m*, one dose.

Bronchitis: chest full of moist râles. Child has suffered from crops of boils and dry scalp eruptions off and on, practically continuously, since birth.

One month later: No return of cough which cleared up very quickly, 'almost instantaneously after your powder', mother reported. Skin is much clearer.

Woman, aged 25. Coryza, sore throat, tonsils swollen and congested; no appetite; feels ill and feverish. Temperature 102°. Pulse 120.

Face red and hot. Cold and chilly and shivery, must sit over the fire, followed by heat and sweat, but still feels shivers coming on when moving or taking bedclothes off; feels very irritable and snappy; cannot speak a decent word to anybody.

Nux vom. cm., one dose, given at 8 p.m. Temperature

down next morning. All symptoms cleared up like magic; patient was able to travel to the south of England from London in the afternoon without feeling any the worse for it and came back a week later to report how well she felt.

Woman, aged 33. Cough and cold in head for a week. Very deaf ever since cold started, both ears were syringed and a quantity of impacted cerumen was removed without improving deafness. Exact symptoms were then taken: frontal and occipital headaches, 'awful throbbing headaches', which are worse stooping and worse motion, worse coughing, cough worse evenings, unable to sleep; mouth dry, very thirsty, 'could drink a bucket of water at a time'.

Weather changeable, warm and wet one day; cold and dry the next day. Patient feels cross and irritable. *Bryonia* 30, a dose three times daily.

Patient came to report herself in three days' time: 'I am well, thank you, and do not want any more medicine. Those powders took my headache straight away.' She did not even ask for a bottle of 'tonic' and volunteered the information that she had never got over so severe a cold so quickly before.

CHRONIC HOARSENESS

The other day quite unexpectedly I was faced with a problem which, but for homoeopathy, I should have been quite unable to deal with. A young man turned up when it was nearly dusk, almost voiceless; in a whisper he informed me his mother had sent him. He had lost his voice over six weeks ago, had been to his own doctor who, after treating him for a week or so, had sent him on to a laryngologist, a specialist for larynx trouble. He had seen him two or three times and as his voice was rather worse than better, he had been told to wait for admission to hospital for further investigations. He rather dreaded this ordeal and felt he would never get his voice back again. It did not hurt him to speak, he simply could not raise his voice above a hoarse whisper.

The rubric, 'painless loss of voice' in Kent's *Repertory* only shows eight remedies, so my search was not a very difficult or lengthy one. The history he gave was that he fell into a ditch full of water about seven weeks ago, when he had been running and was over-heated and perspiring freely. He was able to change his clothes very quickly and yet within twenty-four hours his voice had disappeared. Since then he had been perspiring much too freely, which was quite new to him; he was continually breaking out in violent perspirations. Always very thirsty and had a great desire for cold water. There was a feeling as if he had plenty of mucus in his larynx and if he could only clear his throat he would feel better.

He felt the heat very much and was very fond of sugar — there was also a history of glands of the neck when a child.

Another interesting point which came out on closer inquiry was that he had had eczema recently in the spring, a skin eruption in the right axilla and on the right arm, which had been suppressed with ointments after several weeks treatment. His breath was offensive and putrid, and I found out that he was subject to constipation. His arms were perspiring so freely that he could feel the sweat dripping off him. On all these symptoms, profuse clammy perspiration, painless loss of voice, terrific irritation of skin under shoulders and armpit which was made worse by scratching, great thirst for cold water, I prescribed *Phosphorus* 30.

Three days later he visited me again and I found his voice much stronger; he could speak well above a whisper now. The profuse perspiration had stopped and his usual thirst for large quantities of cold water had gone as well. He felt better in himself and his breath was quite sweet. Notice please, he had not been ordered any aperients or mouthwash. He had been advised to inhale plain steam at night before going to bed. By the bye I forgot to mention he had been ordered medicinal inhalations by his previous doctors without the slightest benefit. *Phos.* 30 was repeated three days later; within six days, on his third visit, his voice was loud and quite tuneful, the natural pitch and timbre was returning. He was delighted, of course, and was returning to work the next day. The following week his voice was absolutely normal.

This was what Homoeopathy can do: voiceless over six

weeks, even a specialist could do nothing without hospital-ization, and as soon as the correct homoeopathic medicine was given in minutest doses, the voice returned, as if by charm. His mother asked 'But why could Mr. – , the specialist, not do the same?' Ask me another. It is because they have not got the key to unlock the treasure house of rational medicinal treatment.

Alas for them and the poor patients who go on attending the hospital departments week after week, sometimes with but little improvement. Of course this young man's diet was altered, he was taken off white bread, put on wholemeal bread, bran, daily fruit and properly cooked vegetables and salads.

A triumph for homoeopathy, do you not agree?

I remember a woman who was voiceless for twelve months; she was suspected of T.B., and had attended a tuberculosis dispensary and ear and throat department of a big teaching hospital for weeks. I had no time to deal with her myself, as it was a children's clinic, so I sent her up to the Homo-eopathic Hospital and within 2-3 weeks her voice came back! I saw her off and on for nearly two years afterwards and her voice remained strong and hearty all through that time. Give me homoeopathy even for such specialized complaints as voice trouble. It does much better than orthodox medicine in functional troubles. And how often is not the patient told, as my two patients mentioned previously, that no cause could be found for the hoarseness.

CHAPTER SIX

SOME ACUTE CONDITIONS

PTOMAINE POISONING?

Awakened by loud ringing of telephone about 3 a.m. An agitated voice at the other end of the wire reported feeling extremely ill, with sensation of impending death, shaking and trembling of muscles — one could hear the chattering of the teeth and the shaking of the 'phone — there was heat of the body, much heat of the lower extremities. No cause could be given for this sudden attack, which roused the patient from a deep sleep. Ptomaine poisoning was considered but, even though mushrooms had been partaken of the previous night, the other members of the family were not struck down: there was no vomiting or diarrhoea. The remedy lay between *Aconite* and *Arsenic*; but *Aconite* won the day, as one remembered the suddenness of the attack, the fact that the patient was a plethoric, strong, well-developed individual, somewhat choleric — and the day before had been cold, dry, and somewhat windy. *Aconite* 30 was prescribed over the 'phone, to be taken at 10 to 15 minutes interval. Result: no further disturbance during the night; patient went to sleep in about two hours' time and was able to go to work by 8.30 in the morning, none the worse for this unpleasant experience. Pathological diagnosis was impossible and unnecessary, as diagnosis of the required indicated remedy was immediate and the disease process was cut short.

ABDOMINAL COLIC

(2) Another nocturnal *dénouement*. Patient was suddenly wakened shortly after midnight by acute abdominal colic and nausea, could hardly get out of bed quick enough in order to get to the lavatory with simultaneous explosion at both ends. Vomiting of extremely bitter bile and loose most offensive

diarrhoea: it was as if a tap was turned on, and there was no holding back. This happened two or three times, accompanied by great prostration, restlessness and anguish, feeling as if the end was near. *Arsenic* 1*m*, given and repeated two or three times at short intervals, and the attacks ceased as suddenly as they had come on, thanks to the efficiency of the correctly given medicine. The choice of this remedy was made easy, as it was remembered that the previous afternoon at a well-known restaurant, ice-cream and cream cakes had been on the menu: and diarrhoea after ice-cream points to *Arsenic*. There was no recurrence of this acute gastro-enteritis. The patient wisely starved for twenty-four hours to give the inflamed mucous membranes of stomach and intestines a good rest.

(3) Called out before 8 a.m. Found young woman writhing in bed with acute abdominal colic and stitching, burning pains: The pains were so severe she wanted to move, but every movement made her shriek out; she had to lie still with the knees drawn up to relax the abdominal muscles; she did not want to be touched, every breath she took made the pain worse. She was asking for cold water, which she would gulp down in big mouthfuls. They were newly married, and the poor husband stood by holding her hand, absolutely helpless and worked up. On examination one found the typical signs of an acute appendicitis: the attack had come on during the early hours of the night; the temperature was 100°, pulse 100-110. One wondered about operation and admitting the patient to hospital, but decided to give Homoeopathy a chance. The patient's symptoms called out for *Bryonia*, and *Bryonia* 1*m* given half-hourly relieved so quickly that after two doses the abdominal muscles relaxed, and by 11 a.m., two hours after she had the first dose, she was sound asleep, the temperature and pulse were normal and the attack was over. She was seen the next day perfectly recovered, happy and smiling. What a godsend Homoeopathy is! The family and the patient were saved the agitation of removal to hospital, the anxiety of a more or less serious operation, followed by several weeks of convalescence, let alone the

expense of it all. She was subsequently given a diet sheet, warned about constipation, forbidden to take irritating laxatives, and three years later there had been no return of any acute abdominal trouble.

GALL-BLADDER COLIC

(4) A young woman, aged 18, came on November 23rd, 1936, complaining of recurrent attacks of gall-bladder colic with jaundice and vomiting; had three attacks since birth of child; attacks every three to four weeks. Said she never had a day's illness until she became pregnant; jaundice and sickness developed some time before child was born. She was kept in hospital for three weeks as she was so ill; they X-rayed her three times and sent her out with the diagnosis, obstruction of gall-bladder, and a very strict diet — no fat, no butter, skimmed milk, fish, etc., to which she stuck religiously, and yet the attacks recurred.

A few more exact symptoms were elicited, such as pains recurred every night, hammering right-sided pains, region of gall-bladder extending through to right shoulder-blade, restless with pain, sits bent over with pain, has to hold herself. This suggested *Chelidonium*; on the other hand there was a great craving for fat (*Ars., Hep.,* NIT.-AC., *Nux v.* and *Sulph.*) and a desire for sweets which left Ars., Nux v. and SULPH. — *Sulphur* being indicated in the highest degree. Mentally she was a Sulphur patient, too; intelligent, inquisitive, wanted to know the why and wherefore of everything — a typical know-all, argumentative philosopher. *Sulphur* 30 was decided on. A week later the report was, ever so much better, no further attacks of pain or jaundice. On December 11th, reported that she could not resist a good helping of suet-pudding three or four days previously, had some pain and retching for four hours, but the attack passed off quickly and there was no jaundice. *Sulphur* 6 night and morning prescribed, as *Sulphur* 30 did not hold long enough. December 21st — no more pains, no jaundice, 'feeling ever so well in herself, has not felt so well for months', has not had any period since baby was born, wondered whether she was pregnant again. *Sulphur* 6 night and morning to be continued.

January 4th, 1937 — very well, no further attacks, has been on ordinary diet, the period came on Christmas Day. Wants to know what the medicine was and wonders why the hospital could not have given her the same simple pills that cured her so quickly. A *Sulphur* patient is an eternal question mark and wants to probe into everything. Is very grateful for having been saved further lengthy examinations and investigations and a threatened operation and insists on taking a further supply of pills with her, so that she can keep them by her in case of another attack.

VOMITING OF LATE PREGNANCY
February, 1916. Woman, seventh pregnancy. Said to be eight months pregnant. Incessant vomiting for the past three weeks, could not keep anything down, not even liquids. Been under allopathic treatment for it; very constipated.

Vomit: dark green, offensive, taste bitter. Prostrated, exhausted, face looked drawn, of an earthy, dirty-greyish colour; eyes dull, sclerotics yellow; tongue dirty grey deposit; teeth carious; breath offensive. Whole patient was offensive and smell was almost putrid, she was evidently toxic. Cold, clammy sweat on forehead. No temperature. Pulse feeble; 96.

Pain in epigastrium, burning in character. Stomach not dilated. Abdomen: no sign of peritonitis. Uterus enlarged to nearly full time; no evidence of labour. Breech presentation.

Symptoms: Patient thirsty, desired small sips of water frequently. Cold, wanted to be covered up; supposed to have been restless at beginning of illness. All these symptoms combined with remarkable foetor and prostration made me think of *Ars.* which was given. Called again three hours later as 'patient was very bad'. Found labour had set in; the baby was born and the second arrived a few minutes after my arrival. Mother still vomiting.

Next morning found practically the same state of affairs. No cessation of vomiting yet. On close questioning I discovered patient craved for *cold water*, which they would not give her for fear of harming her; also severe frontal headache which was relieved only by cold compresses.

Here were all the symptoms of *Phosphorus* and one dose of *Phos.* 10*m* was given plus repeated doses of .S.V.R. Returning 12 hours later, I found the patient cheerful, wonderfully improved. 'No more sickness since the powder you gave me this morning. I enjoyed a cup of tea this afternoon and slept for nearly three hours.' The first unbroken sleep for days.

The next day, patient had a boiled egg for breakfast before my arrival and enjoyed it. The foetor was disappearing fast; the skin had lost its earthy hue. 'But I have such a sore tongue.' On examining her mouth, I found the under surface of tongue practically one big ulcer. This cleared up in two or three days. Breasts began to secrete normally, and the puerperium was uneventful, except that the father was shocked at the arrival of two strangers instead of one.

On going through my desk I found these notes on some of my earlier cases, when I first started out in private practice. Indeed the rapid cure of the case of pernicious vomiting of pregnancy established me in that neighbourhood. The news of it spread like wild-fire. I was venturesome in those days and gave much higher potencies than I do now; I do think that the high and highest potencies work well in acute illnesses, more rapidly than the low potencies, but you have to know your remedies, and you have to be careful not to repeat too soon. In treating chronic diseases, medium potencies are safer in women, who are most sensitive to the action of medicines and the reactions of high potencies and the storms they set up are so violent that few people would have the patience to put up with the extra suffering. In my time I have seen severe disturbances following a dose of a high potency, sometimes most alarming, so I have learnt to play safe.

You will notice too that in 1916 the price of Rectified Spirits of Wine was still within the reach of the pockets of a young doctor who had her living to earn without spare cash, now we should have to use a different kind of non-medicated

Placebo.

One wonders what would happen if the majority of the doctors were homoeopaths! Many acute illnesses would be cut short, there would be less hospital beds required, fewer operations, public money would be saved, and valuable lives would be prolonged. Shall we ever see the day of Homoeopathy being preached from the house tops and taught in all the medical schools?

CHAPTER SEVEN

THE VALUE OF ACONITE

There are no specifics in Homoeopathy. You do not prescribe for the disease, you prescribe for the individual in question. This is a great stumbling-block to both doctors and lay people. On the one hand we get asked over and over again: 'What do you give for a cold, or for bronchitis, or for rheumatism?' — just to mention a few of the commoner complaints. And one has to answer, 'It depends on the patient.' On the other hand, because we consider the individual and do not prescribe according to the name of the disease, we get the reputation of not making a diagnosis. Diagnosis is necessary, always, though it does not help very much in finding a remedy, at least not in all cases. Let me elucidate.

A friend of mine was telling me that her grandfather was a homoeopathic doctor, and they still followed some of his instructions; such as, they always took *Aconite* in small doses for a cold. This is prescribing for a disease, and therefore not homoeopathy. It is not the small dose which makes a medicine homoeopathic to the disease; the question always should be asked: 'Is the medicine or medicines *similar* to the kind of patient afflicted with this disease?'

Aconite sometimes is the simillimum for a certain kind of cold; but there are a number of other medicines which are frequently necessary and indicated for a chill and its effects, and in order to treat them, you have to consider the kind of weather which prevailed when the patient caught his cold, whether wet or dry, cold or hot, windy and stormy. It all makes a difference.

I came across a book on homoeopathic treatment, published 100 years ago, which clearly showed that the earlier homoeopaths, at any rate in England, relied largely on

Aconite for the early treatment of all acute diseases. It did not invariably stop or abort the disease; they had to go on giving other remedies to follow up; the disease seemed to progress, in spite of *Aconite*. The routine treatment seemed to be, whether it was pneumonia, or typhus — just to mention at random two diseases common then — *Aconite* followed by *Bryonia*, or alternating with *Bryonia* or a similar acute remedy. There was no difference as regards the duration of the disease from the ordinary orthodox treatment in this kind of haphazard routine method of prescribing remedies for names of diseases; the death rate was decidedly lower, less harm was done to the patient, it is true, which was an advantage, but it was not and never will be true, or the best homoeopathy.

And again very few people can or do understand why we say that a certain medicine can and does cure different kinds of diseases. We are considered quacks because we prescribe, say, *Bryonia* for rheumatism, bronchitis, pleurisy, constipation, gastric disturbance, hepatic chill, etc., just to mention one remedy. *Bryonia* may come in for any one of these complaints, but the symptoms necessary for *Bryonia* are what we look for and the identical symptoms may be found in either rheumatism or pneumonia or bronchitis, etc.

Let us return to *Aconite*. I do not very often prescribe *Aconite* for a chill, not in England anyway; but I have found *Aconite* symptoms in a variety of complaints. One very hot summer *Aconite* was always cropping up. During the spell of almost tropical heat, two cases of intussusception in infants round about five to six months were admitted within a day or two. The histories were similar. Each child had been seized with a sudden attack of screaming, great restlessness, the abdomen was distended, which was soon followed by the child passing blood and clear mucus from the back passage. I felt a lump in the right iliac region, the rectum was distended like a balloon when I examined it digitally, and I definitely felt the invaginated piece of bowel high up, and there was this red jelly-like substance oozing from the rectum. I gave the No. 1 child two doses of *Aconite m* at fifteen minutes' interval, the intussusception disappeared and there was no need for any operation. The child was kept in for observation for several days, but there was no need to repeat the medicine, nor was the surgeon required.

Child No. 2 was seen by the surgeon on admission, as he was on the spot; he made the diagnosis. While we were waiting to get the infant into the theatre, I gave him two doses of *Aconite m*, and when the surgeon re-examined him on the operating table, he could find no sign of any intussusception. The bowel had slipped back in the interval after the *Aconite*, and the surgeon decided not to operate. I told him, then, I had given the *Aconite* as it had cleared up a similar condition two days previously. The temperature outside was very high, tropical in fact. He was astonished how quickly the medicine had acted.

The symptoms indicating *Aconite* in bowel troubles are passage of pure, bright red blood and mucus, with tenesmus, with high fever which comes on suddenly in well-developed, active, healthy children in hot weather. Great restlessness, anguish and much screaming with pain.

I saw another infant about that time. She passed light green motions with much restlessness, her face was red, her eyes were glassy, her temperature was 104°, a typical case of summer diarrhoea. A few doses of *Aconite m* and the diarrhoea disappeared, the temperature dropped to normal, and the storm was over. Within twenty-four hours everything had cleared up.

Bowel troubles like these are apt to come on in hot summer; and are frequently found in tropical countries. Here the disease would be called Dysentery, and bacteriologically you might find the particular *Bacillus Dysentericus* or the 'Sonne' *Bacillus*. But I am quite sure that *Aconite* would have cleared up a certain percentage of the dysentery cases which occurred in Mesopotamia during the 1914-18 War, and it will always cure rapidly a large number of dysentery cases in the tropics, or in any other country during a hot spell.

There is another totally different set of circumstances which call for *Aconite*, and that is intensely cold winds; or cold wind combined with snow. I saw several children this spring suffering from bronchitis which cleared up with a few doses of *Aconite*. One child I remember, I was sent for some years ago; the parents were in a great state about him; he was a fair, chubby child, he had been playing about in an icy cold wind the day before, and in the night he was suddenly seized with a dry barking cough, high fever, somewhere round about 103°. He was restless, frightened, the throat and larynx burned and he asked for cold water and could hardly swallow it. It was an attack of croup or acute laryngitis; but a few doses of *Aconite* soon set him right; he was well in a day and there was no return of the trouble.

This reminds me of another case of croup which always came on after exposure to a cold east wind. He was wakened night after night with a constant dry, barking cough; usually it came on after midnight. The child was five years old, he had been taken to various hospitals and doctors, had swallowed a great many bottles of medicine — with no effect. Whenever there was an east wind, the child developed laryngitis and bronchitis. The mother brought him to me for an overhaul before going to school. I gave him — not *Aconite* this time — *Aconite* has not got this constantly recurring condition: cough coming on night after night, waking him up in the latter part of the night; he was not restless and anguished enough for *Aconite*. No, I gave him *Hepar sulph.*, one powder high, I think it was the 1,000th potency — and promptly forgot about him. I did not hear anything more of the child until six or seven years later, when the mother turned up with another baby. The first thing she said to me: 'Do you remember, doctor, the powder you gave to Harry for his croup when he was five years old; he has never had another attack of croup since, he can go out in all kinds of weather, wind does not effect him any more. He is perfectly well.' If I had given him *Aconite*, on the diagnosis: croup after exposure to cold wind, I should have failed in this case; it was a *Hepar* case and *Hepar* cured him miraculously and at once.

I had another patient, an old lady this time. It was a cold

spring again; she was very sensitive to cold winds, and she got a chill on the bladder quite suddenly; burning pains in the bladder, cutting, sharp pains with hot, scalding urine — which was bright red in colour, and contained blood. She was always sitting on the commode and straining and straining to pass water. Extremely restless and frightened, so frightened, she *knew* she was going to die, so that she sent for the whole family, and they all of them arrived promptly, sons and daughters and grandchildren, to see the old lady pass away. Only it did not come off, for a few doses of *Aconite* had been given her, and the cystitis stopped, the pain and the urging went, and also the fear of death. And the old lady — she was seventy-five years at least — survived for several years.

Death was cheated by a few minute doses of *Aconite*.

Have I made myself clear? *Aconite* is not a panacea for all evils. Homoeopathy is not quackery, we have a scientific law, which says 'Like cures like'. *Aconite* taken in material doses produces these symptoms of anguish, restlessness, fever, heat, thirst, in the healthy person, and if you give *Aconite* when you find these same symptoms in the sick, you will cure cases of diarrhoea, dysentery, intussusception, croup, bronchitis, pneumonia, cystitis and others — instantly. But do not prescribe *Aconite* for every case of chill or cold; it will fail you, unless you know the indications. So it is with every remedy. Treat the patient and not the disease; this is the great principle in Homoeopathy.

Let me recapitulate. *Aconite* is a fine remedy, it does cut short diseases, when it is indicated, but it has no periodicity; it is of no use in a continuous fever, or in an intermittent one. It is short-acting, quick in its action. *Aconite* is not homoeopathic or similar to every rise of temperature or pyrexia as such. How easy homoeopathy would be if we had little pigeon-holes for diseases and their respective remedies.

CHAPTER EIGHT

ABDOMINAL UPSETS OF EVERYDAY LIFE

We are told that Homoeopathy is based on the law that 'like cures like'. How does this law work out in practice in acute cases?

There is the *Ipecacuanha* case. It is well known that *Ipecac* produces vomiting, has an emetic effect in large doses. This is the physiological effect, therefore, if the statement as promulgated by Samuel Hahnemann is correct, *Ipecac.* in small doses should be curative in cases where vomiting is the prominent symptom. But nausea and vomiting is a common symptom in gastric disturbances, and if you gave *Ipecac.* in all cases of sickness, you might hit it sometimes, but many times you would miss and find it would not work. Do not say then that Homoeopathy is not of any use because it failed you. It failed because prescribing on one symptom alone is not sufficient; always look for the three-legged stool, on which to base a homoeopathic prescription — try and find at least three symptoms which point to a particular remedy.

Let me illustrate this by a case which happened to me a little while ago. I was called in a great hurry and the message was that the patient was continually vomiting. I packed half a dozen remedies and went to see her. I found the patient collapsed and prostrate, she had been vomiting for a little over an hour and had brought up quantities of bile-stained fluid, there was constant nausea and pain in the pit of the stomach, vomiting brought no relief. Even while I was there, she started to retch and complained of this distressing nausea. Her face looked grey and drawn, the pulse was feeble, 68 per minute, and the temperature did not reach 96° Fahrenheit, she was suffering from collapse and felt cold to the touch. The tongue was clean, in spite of the nausea and vomiting; in cases of vomiting the tongue is coated as a rule. This attack had come on after exposure to a cold east wind the previous day. I gave *Ipecacuanha* at once and stayed to watch the effect.

Within less than five minutes, the greyness of the complexion disappeared, the pink flush came back, the eyes brightened, the face was less drawn and instead of moaning 'I feel so sick', she began to smile and take an interest in some social event which was much talked of in the papers at the moment. There was no further sickness while I was in the house; the vomiting had been continuous for well over an hour beforehand, as I said previously. I rang up three hours later, and the report was that the patient was comfortable and had been asleep and the vomiting had stopped completely. She continued taking the *Ipecac.* four-hourly for twelve hours, and had no return of nausea or vomiting. It completely stopped after the first dose of *Ipecac.* The symptoms on which I prescribed *Ipecacuanha* were: nausea and vomiting without relief, clean tongue, collapse and faintness, and colicky, stabbing pains in the region of the stomach.

The three most important symptoms were overwhelming nausea with clean tongue and vomiting without relief, and prostration.

Allopathically the correct thing to give would have been a bismuth and soda bicarbonate mixture, with some Acid Hydrocyanicum to ease the pain. I do not remember ever having seen such instantaneous relief after a bismuth mixture in the early days when I followed the orthodox methods — such quick results, as I got after a simple, small pellet of *Ipecacuanha* in the 1,000th potency. Such a high potency is not necessary, a dose of *Ipecacuanha* in the third decimal, or 3*x*, would have worked just as well, only I happened to have this potency, the 1*m* or 1,000th potency with me. Hahnemann himself preferred to work with fairly high potencies, medicines which were prepared or potentized — made more potent by an exact and precise mode of preparation, according to a definite scale. This scale of dilution was 1 in 100, small quantities of original drug substance were used each time and carefully measured and carefully triturated, for a definite length of time, if a solid drug. If liquid, the drug was succussed or shaken up by hand with the diluent, either alcohol or alcohol and water for a definite length of time. This produced the first potency, or 1c — the C being the Roman symbol for 100 — one drop of the first potency with 99 drops of diluent, *well shaken*, produced the second potency and so on, step by step until the higher potencies are reached — the 30th or higher still.

The decimal scale was introduced later; each step in the series of potentization being one-tenth of the previous potency, so that 3x, or the third decimal strength, contained one-thousandth of the drug power or drug substance, and 6x contained one millionth of the drug. This strength was not obtained by just diluting it, by putting one drop in nearly 2.1 ounces of water — which is 1 in 1,000,000, but by diluting small quantities each time in six stages. As I said before, the lower potencies, such as 3x or 6x are safer potencies to use for beginners, either lay or professional. The higher potencies should be left for the use of more experienced doctors.

Having discussed potencies, let us go back to clinical cases and remedies for acute digestive disturbances.

A lady I knew had dined not wisely but too well at a 3-course dinner, followed an hour later by weak China tea. Three hours afterwards she noticed great distension and fullness of the abdomen, obstructed flatulence which could not be dispersed. There was a feeling of weight in the gastric region and difficulty in breathing, nausea with retching, colicky pains with urging to stool and straining to pass a scanty stool. Coldness and shivering and anxiety.

One dose of *Nux vom.* brought an explosion of wind and a diarrhoeic stool, pale and white in colour, showing a liver upset, after which there was peace, the abdomen became flat and the patient went to sleep at once. The acute dyspepsia cleared up in ten minutes and there was no need for any further medication. One dose was sufficient.

In both these cases the indicated remedy aborted the attacks. The acute chill was cured at once in the first case by

Ipecacuanha, the acute dyspepsia caused by rich food in a sedentary person was at once antidoted by *Nux vomica*, and the disease processes were prevented from extending further.

Let us see whether Homoeopathy works also when the acute disease has lasted for several days. A boy just over six years of age was brought to me in January, 1938, with a history of diarrhoea of ten days' duration, which came on after a chill. He was by this time deeply jaundiced, eyes yellow, complexion sallow, deep rings under the eyes, the motions were white, and the urine thick and deeply pigmented, and showed the colour reaction produced by bile salts. He was very thirsty for warm drinks, tongue coated thickly with white fur, felt worse after eating; he had pains in the abdomen specially in the liver and gall bladder region, which were improved by firm pressure. He could not take a deep breath without bringing on a cutting, stitching pain in his right side. The symptoms called so plainly for *Bryonia*, that he was given *Bryonia* 30, which he was ordered to take three times a day. He was put on a fat-free diet, dry toast, without butter, skimmed milk and water, barley water, and I saw him three days later and heard that the diarrhoea had stopped the same day, the motions twenty-four hours later were the usual brown colour; on examinationn the eyes were clear, no jaundice anywhere, the urine was clear, straw colour, and showed an acid reaction. The urine had cleared in two days.

Homoeopathy and the correctly indicated remedy had worked again, rapidly, painlessly and efficiently, even though the child had been ill for ten days. Perhaps, you will say, the disease had worked itself out by the time the boy came. Granted, there might be something in this, only why was it, that for ten days the boy was steadily getting worse, and as soon as he began to take *Bryonia*, the jaundice and the diarrhoea cleared up in a few hours, in just over a day or barely two days? One swallow does not make a summer; but if a Homoeopath gets case after case where the correct — mind you, it must be correct — remedy, the remedy which produced similar symptoms in the healthy — cures the sick person, he can only continue to affirm that he is right, and that the cure is not accidental, but due to the medicine.

My mind flashes back along the vista of years, and I recall a case of acute jaundice in a doctor friend of mine, a newly qualified man who was house-surgeon at that time to a well-known physician at the large hospital where I received my training. I was still a student in those days. This young doctor surely should have had, you would have thought, the best of scientific advice from the famous professor he worked under. He was ordered daily doses of calomel, followed by morning doses of epsom salts; he was put on a starvation, strictly fat-free diet. I was staying in the same house and saw him daily, and watched the misery he was in. Irritable, grouchy to the last degree, could not be spoken to without snapping the other person's head off. He was apparently suffering from the cold, as he was always sitting crouched over the fire; he was a studious fellow and did not go in for exercise at all. These were the things I noticed, and now I should know what to give him, in order to cut short the attack of jaundice, I should give him *Nux vomica* and should guarantee a cure in twenty-four to forty-eight hours. This young doctor, full of the most scientific lore, and carrying out the instructions of his teacher, took well over fourteen days, nearly three weeks, before he was quite recovered! It was an obstinate attack and he was run down after too much study, I was told then, and I believed it, still being in the apprentice stage.

Years afterwards, when I had imbibed of the milk of Homoeopathy, I came across a similar case. This was a middle-aged man who had recently joined the masonic fraternity and had to partake of the dinners which go with their ceremonies. He always came to me the day after such a dinner with an early attack of jaundice, yellowish eyes, dirty skin, showing a coated, foul tongue, worse in the morning, with bursting headaches, feeling as if there was a stone in the chest and such a vile temper; his wife and his employees used to dread these days after the night before. He could not digest the rich food and his liver certainly did not take kindly to the wine and the alcoholic drinks.

Nux vomica 30, three or four times a day set him right in approximately twenty-four hours, but I could not persuade him to give up his masonic dinners and specially the drinks. 'Anyway,' he said, 'you are the gainer, as I have to come to you to get me well of my liver and very quickly your medicine acts, too.' His wife was thankful also, for the *Nux vom.* used to cure him rapidly of his irritability and his liver.

The *Nux vom.* patient is a gourmet, he likes good food, but he cannot eat much, his digestion is easily upset and his liver gets easily disordered by the richness of the particular kind of food he likes.

Bryonia on the other hand is a gourmand; he does not mind what he eats, it is the quantity he is after, a ravenous eater, who is made ill by eating too much.

They both get jaundiced after an attack of anger. *Nux vom.*, feels so angry that he has a desire to stab the person who makes him angry, he is particularly angry and irritable in the mornings, so do not tackle a *Nux vom.* person in the morning. *Bryonia*, on the other hand, loses his temper and gets more angry in the evening. *Bryonia* is very thirsty with his liver and stomach complaints, *Nux vom.* is not thirsty. *Bryonia* is worse from motion and better firm pressure, *Nux vom.* is worse from slightest pressure and worse motion, and has constant and repeated calls to go to stool, a feeling as if he was never done.

In this way you individualize and particularize each remedy, and thus an acute illness will be cut short rapidly, if the right remedy is recognised and applied.

Another very common jaundice remedy is *Chelidonium*, the Greater Celandine. This plant is well known among the herbalists and Galen and Dioscorides hundreds of years ago prescribed it for jaundice, probably on the theory of 'signatures'. The claim was that the bile-like juice of *Chelidonium* and the yellow flowers, pointed the way to the disease it could cure. And apparently on broad indications in large doses it does act as an organ remedy and is very helpful in some liver affections.

It has been proved homoeopathically on healthy individuals and it certainly produces symptoms which point to the liver as being the chief organ affected by it, and therefore it is curative in all sorts of maladies, where the liver is involved as well.

I remember a young man, a carpenter by trade, who for some unknown reason developed jaundice. He complained chiefly of a continuous aching pain at the lower angle of the right scapula or shoulder blade. He was sitting up in bed, bent forward on his elbows, unable to move with the acute stabbing it produced whenever he tried to change his position. Creeping chilliness and nausea and vomiting, and only hot, almost boiling water, would stay down. He was bothered with diarrhoea and the motions were bright yellow. In fact everything was yellow, his tongue was thickly coated and yellow, with a narrow red margin. His skin and eyes were yellow and his behaviour and outlook were yellow and jaundiced. Two or three doses of *Chelidonium* 30 in thirty-six hours cleared up his malaise, his vomiting, and he was back at work in three days.

The first sign of indisposition his wife had noticed was his dislike for cheese, of which he was inordinately fond and he would always order it for his supper, as a rule. A small abnormality like this would mean nothing to the allopathic physician, but to the homoeopath this dislike of cheese with the other symptoms, pointed to *Chelidonium*, and it disposed of the illness rapidly.

There are many other remedies for biliousness, each one with its own peculiar indications. As it has been pointed out again and again in these pages, the name of the disease, the diagnosis is of secondary importance, consider the patient, his idiosyncrasies, the changes from the normal, such as sudden distaste to cheese, vomiting relieved by hot drinks, and pain underneath the angle of the right scapula, or pain going through from front to back in the region of the liver; this combination of symptoms calls for *Chelidonium*, as I have said.

Bryonia shows slightly different symptoms. *Nux vomica*

has a set of different symptoms. *Lycopodium* is different again. Find the right combination, apply the suitable remedy and you will get a rapid cure.

Belladonna may cure a patient with gallstone colic, the picture he presents would be as follows: in bed with extreme heat, and sensitiveness, cannot bear to be touched, or have the bed jarred, screams with pain, face red and hot; *Bell.* in a few minutes will relieve such a one.

There are many remedies for jaundice, for biliousness, for gallstone colic, etc., the best thing for a physician in all acute cases, is to memorize the symptoms of the more common drugs for each complaint so that he can recognize and distinguish the China case of biliousness from the *Natrum sulph.* or the *Mercury* case say, just to mention two or three which may be necessary. Such books as Allen's Materia Medica or Nash's Materia Medica or Tyler's Drug Pictures are most valuable in learning, comparing and contrasting the various remedies. If you have made friends with each one of the commoner, more frequently used drugs, you will find it not too difficult to recognize a drug at the bed-side.

Acute diseases, even though they are frequently self-limited and have a tendency to get well of themselves, do get definitely such a stimulus from the right remedy, applied according to the Law of Similars that the disease seems to disappear in a few hours.

CHAPTER NINE

TWO OUT-PATIENT CASES

The out-patients hall is full, a subdued hum of voices is heard from the crowd who, while waiting for the doctor's bell, are discussing one another's ailments and comparing notes with great relish; the more lurid the details, the more they enjoy it. An afternoon's out-patients means strenuous work for the doctor; a quick summing up as each patient enters, a rapid switching over from one serious problem to another, a snap diagnosis after a more or less thorough examination, and then the quickest part of the interview for the orthodox physician, the writing down of the stock mixture for the inevitable bottle of medicine which is the patient's delight — while if necessary the name is entered on the ever lengthening list for admission for further investigation and maybe an operation.

The task is made much more difficult for the homoeopath; there are no stock mixtures, each patient has to have individual attention and the indicated medicine should be found, which will ease the complaint and more than likely cure it. The doctor must have a prodigious memory; there are certainly textbooks and repertories at hand, but you cannot spend much time searching through repertories while scores of patients are waiting.

You may not get any startling cures in out-patients' work; time is too short, but much useful work can be done and is done in dispensary and hospital out-patients; and cases are cured by homoeopaths which have had months or even years of treatment by the orthodox school. Let me give examples of this kind who happened to turn up on the same day.

One of the first was a woman of 55 who had been a collar hand in a large outfitter's store for years. Unfortunately for her the menopause gave her much trouble and in spite of the panel doctor's administrations, reinforced by frequent visits to hospital, she did not get better, and though she tried hard to go on working and made several valiant attempts to return to the work-room, she always collapsed when she got there, and, in the end, she had been existing for several years on the panel insurance money. She would have starved of course on this pitiful allowance, if she had not lived with friends. A very kind charitable lady also allowed her a small pension to augment her income.

A tall angular woman, grey-haired, indecisive, slow of speech, blushing furiously when addressed by a stranger, specially a doctor; frightened and scared of doctors, says they cannot do her any good, has seen so many and none could help her. Can hardly walk the half mile from her room to the dispensary without resting several times. The walk made the palpitations of the heart much worse, these palpitations were her main trouble, they come on with any exertion, they wake her during the night, and they may continue for hours. The other trouble which is nearly as bad are the heat paroxysms which she gets. She cannot stand any heat, any close room is too much for her. The main reason why she had to give up work was she could not sit in the work-room as this brought on terrible flushes and heats and palpitations. She cannot bear a fire in the room, it makes her go all hot and bothered. She has got the 'eiderdown complex' very strongly marked, that is: she cannot bear any warm clothes on her bed, she used to share a double bed with her friend, but had to give it up and take to a camp bed, as the friend liked warm clothes, blankets and an eiderdown on the bed, and she could only bear the lightest of sheets and blankets over her. She could not bear any tight clothes round her waist, nor any high-necked blouses or frocks, these nearly choked her. Her complexion was bluish, cyanosed cheeks and lips, there was perspiration on her face which felt hot to the touch, the hands were hot and moist and trembled on extension. A fine tremor showed on stretching her arms out, the pulse rate was between 110-120, the eyes were not too prominent, but the thyroid gland was slightly enlarged in the middle line, which showed most when she swallowed.

All these symptoms showed that the heart was sound enough, but that too much thyroid was circulating in her blood vessels and interfering with the flow of blood and by constantly disturbing the superficial blood vessels, was causing the superficial heats and attacks of perspiration.

Homoeopathically she was a typical case of *Lachesis*, and she was given *Lachesis* 30 at her first visit. She was seen at fortnightly intervals and kept under the action of *Lachesis* for months. *Eighteen* months have gone by since her first attendance. She can now walk quite briskly without being troubled by palpitations. She sleeps soundly and is hardly ever disturbed or wakened up during the night. She very rarely gets any palpitations during the daytime, and then they only last a short half-hour or so. The pulse rate has gone down to between 60-70 — there are no hot flushes, no perspirations, the hands are cool and do not perspire or tremble any more. The thyroid gland is hardly noticeable. Another problem arises now, or will arise shortly. She is so much better, her mental balance has become so much steadier. What about her returning to work? She has been away from work and on the panel now for over seven years and she has reached the age when she cannot find any new work, and her old job is no longer open to her. The insurance money will soon cease, if and when the insurance doctors find out how much she has improved, fortunately the machine moves slowly. She is a strong argument in favour of pensions for spinsters over 55 years of age. She is well enough to carry on with her normal duties in the house, but will never stand again the stress and strain of rushing to work day after day.

This woman was ill for well over seven years before being seen; she had been seen by many doctors and also surgeons who did not consider her a suitable case for removal of the thyroid; her life was made a misery to her, she was anxious and willing to work, and yet her disabilities would not let her. She was useless and thrown on the scrap-heap in the forties. If she had been given her indicated remedy when she first started to complain, she would have not been off work for very long and would still be a useful member of society. How many others are there like her? Hundreds, probably thousands!

Another case, illustrating the power of the indicated homoeopathic remedy, was seen the same day.

A woman, again in the late forties, presented herself with asthma. She had been cured of asthma and heart by homoeopathy several years ago and had been free of all trouble for three years. In January, 1938, she developed bronchitis, pleurisy and asthma, the usual 'complication of disease' as they call it, and was treated by her panel doctor who came in regularly to her; she was too ill to go out. For months she lay in bed and when she was seen in June, five months after the first day of illness, she still had bronchitis, she still had asthma and still had pains in her chest on taking a deep breath, which she called pleuritic pains, but were not true pleurisy. She was barely able to crawl about again. Her chest was full of asthmatic and bronchial sounds, her breathing was short and laboured, she was deeply cyanosed and blue, she was gasping, her neck muscles were doing overtime as the asthma was bothering her so. I gently scolded her for not coming sooner, and asked her why she had not done so, she had been treated for asthma several years back and had been entirely free of these attacks 'of asthma and heart' – the original diagnosis made by the hospital – for three years. She said she did not like to come back as she had stayed away for so long. I found her asthma troubled her most at night, after midnight, she was restless and agitated, afraid of dying, felt the heat and liked to take sips of warm water. *Arsenic* was her remedy, and *Arsenic* 30 one dose nightly on going to bed was the prescription. She was asked to come back next week, but was not seen again for a month. The asthma had disappeared almost immediately after the *Arsenic* had been given. She felt very well. She looked years younger; her complexion was rosy, her breathing was quiet, no signs of asthma or bronchitis in her chest.

She said she had felt so well since getting the bottle of sugar pills, there was no need for another visit. She only called in that day, as she was passing just to say thank you!

And she had been ill for five months with asthma, bronchitis, pleurisy and heart! and after all these months of sickness a few doses of *Arsenic*, which was the remedy indicated, cleared up this illness of months' standing. Homoeopathy is great and an enormous help in chronic diseases.

These are only two cases seen on one day. There were many such cases of equal interest, perhaps another time I may continue the story.

CHAPTER TEN

LACHESIS IN WOMEN'S DISEASES

A very old lady the other day was telling me about Matthew Duncan who was her doctor many years ago. A very famous man he was in his day; one of the best known women's doctors, and one of the first, if not actually the first, to remove ovaries for all sorts of women's complaints. This was a great undertaking in the eighties and nineties; nowadays it is not thought of very much. More daring and wonderful operations are performed every day; operations on the heart, the lungs, the brain; feats of skill, undreamt of fifty years ago.

I cannot help thinking sometimes that while the skill of the surgeon has improved greatly, the physician is apt to give up too soon and pass on his cases to the surgeon. Such a pity! It gives the homoeopathic physician a great pleasure to be able to cure people without operations, and you may be sure, if a homoeopath recommends an operation, it is absolutely necessary.

Many surgeons remind me of young amateur gardeners who, after having sown seeds, are not content to wait until they come up, but must be continually probing and digging up the earth again, to see what is there.

I am quite sure many young women need never have the operations they are told they must have in order to recover their health, and they would be saved much unnecessary suffering if they had homoeopathic treatment.

Let me relate a case to illustrate how an operation can be prevented.

I had known this young woman for years. She had always been delicate from childhood on, suffered from terrible bouts of constipation and often fainted from pains due to obstinate constipation.

Her periods were just times of acute misery to her; agonizing colicky pains for hours and hours, she used to roll about on the floor with the agony of it, shrieking and shrieking and crying for help, until at last she fainted from sheer exhaustion.

She was a thin slip of a thing, flat like a board, no womanly curves at all; a typical case of ovarian dysfunction and under development.

She was at last seen by a surgeon who diagnosed an ovarian cyst which was removed in due course. There was no relief in her suffering, if anything the bouts of pain got worse and nothing would relieve the constipation except large doses of purgatives. The doctor said this was caused by a displacement of the womb, for which he advised a pessary or uterine support. This she wore for several months and still no change in the suffering. Another operation was proposed, this time it was to be a suspensory operation of the uterus, to cure the prolapsed, retroverted organ. Mind you, she was a young unmarried girl in the twenties! My heart bled when I heard of all the suffering she had been through, and how nothing constructive had been suggested. Her mother at last enquired whether Homoeopathy would or could do anything to prevent any further operations and to cure the agonies of pain she went through every month.

I explained that Homoeopathy was the woman's friend, and I could promise a cure.

I examined and found a retroverted, somewhat enlarged uterus, and a prolapsed, tender left ovary; but so far no recurrence of an ovarian cyst.

She was, as I said, extremely thin, and weighed less than 7 stones. So I advised that she must try and put on weight. She was ordered to drink 1 to 2 pints of milk or buttermilk daily, take extra butter and eggs, plenty of raw salads and fruit and only brown bread instead of white bread. Also oatmeal porridge was prescribed and bran. All this was ordered with a view to cure the constipation.

The next thing that had to be tackled was the premenstrual and early menstrual pain. Here Homoeopathy came in.

I found out on enquiry that her flow was excessive, she passed many dark clots, accompanied with excruciating pains. The odour was very penetrating and unpleasant but, once the clots had passed and the flow had set in properly, the acute pains, which usually came on for four to five days before the periods, ceased completely, and she herself felt much relieved. She was also completely knocked over by warm weather and suffered intensely in the heat, could hardly crawl about in the summer.

Intense headaches before the period, relieved when the period came on.

I saw the remedy as soon as she started to explain her sufferings to me: left-sided pains, dark clots, all her sufferings relieved by the free flow of the menses, and a person much affected by heat, spelt *Lachesis*, and *Lachesis* 30 was prescribed.

I did not see her again for six months, but I had frequent reports, and her mother told of a general all-round improvement. The diet improved the constipation until in quite a short time she required no further laxatives. She had swallowed pints of liquid paraffin and various paraffin emulsions previously. The bowels moved smoothly without any effort and without pain, and she was extremely grateful for this. She found most relief from drinking an infusion of bran sweetened with Barbadoes sugar and flavoured with lemon juice.

As for her periods, she could hardly believe that it was possible she could have no pain, they came along with ease, no suffering beforehand, the clots improved, the colour became normal. She had profuse perspirations previously as well, with a most unpleasant odour. She was very conscious of this and it was impossible sometimes to be in the same room with her. This disappeared also, for which she was almost more grateful than for being relieved from all the pains. When I saw her again, six months after the first visit, she had gained a stone in weight, the uterus was no longer retroverted, and the left ovary no longer tender and prolapsed.

She had some more *Lachesis* 30, which carried her on for a few months. After this she used to come or send for a repetition every few months, whenever there was the slightest return of pains or discomfort. She improved all round; physically as well as mentally; the breasts began to grow and develop, and the curious part was, she had felt previously that however hard she tried, she could never attract a man. Suddenly, however, men began to take an interest in her, asked her to go out to dances with them, and soon she had three or four gentlemen friends who vied with each other to give her a good time. She became happier, more contented in the home, and was a real help to her mother instead of always ailing, always demanding sympathy and attention and nursing.

She religiously kept on the fruit, bran, brown bread and vegetable diet, with plenty of milk and cheese. And so she developed into quite an attractive young woman, full of the joy of living. She was kept on *Lachesis 30, later Lachesis m̄*, and the symptoms always remaining the same, she was put on *Lachesis* 10m.

I only see her at rare intervals now, when she comes for a repetition of the medicine, and each time there is a great improvement in the general physical make-up.

She has had no pains for years, no more constipation, and there is no more talk of an operation. The ovarian cyst has not recurred so far; the surgeon told her mother that there was a small cyst which he left behind as otherwise he would have had to remove both ovaries; and he warned that it would most probably grow and give her trouble later on. The first operation was now well over ten years ago, I think, and for years now she has been quite normal and quite free from pain and menstrual difficulties and sufferings.

Is it not worth while to try Homoeopathy and thus prevent operations?

Lachesis is a remedy derived from a South American snake and should be given in single doses only, spaced at long intervals at least 3-6 months in between each dose, and not below the 30th potency.

Lachesis is not always the remedy for dysmenorrhoea or for cases of ovarian cysts. Other remedies may be necessary, and must be chosen according to the totality of the symptoms, as presented by each patient.

Dysmenorrhoea is a terrible affliction for young girls and can be cured easily. There is no need for a curetting and dilatation of the uterus, no need for morphia and all the pain-killing drugs which have to be taken in ever-increasing doses. Many doctors advise gland treatment nowadays, which is not always successful either; no, the simillimum, the remedy chosen according to the principle that like cures like, is by far and away the best thing to relieve a woman's suffering and prevent the wholesale removal of important organs.

CHAPTER ELEVEN

CONSIDER HOMOEOPATHY BEFORE SURGERY

When I was a house surgeon years ago at a Homoeopathic hospital, I was struck at the number of people who came to be treated in order to avoid operations. Years have gone by and one would have thought that with the vaunted progress in medicine, operative interference would have been less; alas! that this is not so. There are very few people who escape the knife of the surgeon, and indeed the majority do not want to escape, they revel in it, and if you suggest medical treatment, they rather go to somebody else who is sure to advise an operation. Women's diseases are almost entirely dealt with by the surgeon; the physician has been replaced by the surgeon in the majority of the cases.

The homoeopathic physician does not deny that the knife is necessary in some cases to remove an offending organ; but he would explore every avenue first, before he would call in a surgeon. Latterly several people have come my way who have been saved from the surgeon and whose health has been improved enormously at the same time. On May 25th, 1938, a woman in the forties came with the history of bleeding due to a uterine polypus. She was in hospital for three weeks and would have had the operation, only she was too weak to stand it, and was sent out to get strong first. Her uterus was to be removed in a couple of months; in the interval she came for a tonic. She looked very pale and washed out, as people do who have lost much blood. I found the uterus enlarged and bulky, and a small cervical polypus.

I put her on *Fraxinus americana*, the uterine organ remedy of Dr. Burnett's, for a month. The bleeding went on, just a continual ooze. I gave her *Ipecacuanha* 30 for the next acute attack she had, as she felt faint and collapsed, the blood was bright red. The acute haemorrhage was somewhat relieved;

but then the slow oozing started again; she was a person who suffered from flushes and headaches, was extremely loquacious. I could never get her out without a spate of words about nothing; the haemorrhage was now dark, almost black; I thought surely this is *Lachesis*. Again she came two weeks later, with only slight improvement. *Fraxinus americana* three times a day in water to diminish the heavy, congested uterus, was again prescribed. Alas! two weeks afterwards she came in worse than ever; she had been having a severe attack of haemorrhage again, the blood had poured from her, she was collapsed, exsanguinated, her lips were white and bloodless, she looked ghastly. She had been losing heavily for ten days. She was then given *China m*, twelve doses, three times a day, and told to stop the powders when the bleeding ceased. If the bleeding continued, she was to go with a letter to the Homoeopathic Hospital for further treatment, as an operation might be necessary. This was on July 25th, 1938, two months after first coming up for treatment. My holiday was near and I could not look after her in August. I was very grieved and upset, as I was sure her uterus would be out before my return. I saw her again in September, a fresh complexioned smiling woman came bustling in: 'How are you?' I asked — 'you have not had your operation then?' 'Oh, no,' she answered, 'there was no need to go up to hospital after all; the bleeding stopped within twelve hours after I saw you in July, and I have had no return of it; and I only had to take two special powders!'

Two powders of *China* in the 1,000th potency, cleared up the haemorrhage which had troubled her for at least three months! I examined her again, the uterus was nearly normal in size, the polypus had dropped off. She was well again. I see her at regular intervals, the cure holds good. She has her regular periods which last for three to four days, normal in every way, and she has not required any more *China*. No return of the haemorrhage and no return of the uterine polypus.

She tells me everybody comments on her looks; they tell her she is looking so well and so young. 'Yes,' she adds, 'and I did feel half dead when I came here first, now I can work and run about with the youngest without feeling tired.'

She was saved from a severe operation; she is enjoying her life and is grateful to homoeopathy which brought it about.

Allopathically there is no cure for uterine bleeding except heroic doses of ergot; if that does not help a curetting is done, and in middle-aged women the only suggestions are removal of the uterus or artificial menopause brought on by radium. Homoeopathy can do better than this. We have a number of remedies for bleeding; find the right remedy and the bulky, hypertrophied uterus disappears as if by magic.

Unfortunately some doctors will not believe that this is possible and scorn the idea of curing such gynaecological conditions by medicines. I will give you an example of this. A girl in the early thirties was sent to me in July, 1937, for a fibroid, diagnosed as such by a woman surgeon. The patient in question was under a psychologist and this doctor considered an operation bad for the psychological state this girl was in. I found a large uterus with a fibroid in the anterior wall, the size of an orange. I told her I could cure this, provided she was willing to attend regularly.

She came monthly, always full of her psychological conflicts and such like things. I concentrated on her physical condition, the symptoms this self-centred woman presented were of little use to a homoeopath for prescribing; there were pages and pages of them. The mental symptoms in this case were of secondary importance; but the uterine ones were, I considered, of paramount value, and the subsequent history proved I was right. As the uterine condition cleared up, her mental condition cleared as well! She complained largely of extremely painful periods since the age of 13 — she was now 35; they were extremely irregular, came on at five to fourteen weeks' interval, she never knew when to expect them. She would be free for weeks, sometimes once in three months, sometimes two months, sometimes five weeks — they were profuse, she used fifteen or twenty-four towels during the five days; had downbearing pressure, felt very cold, had cold sweats with the pains, had to take veganin for

the pains. Also suffers from actue attacks of palpitations —
tachycardia, which came on without warning. Her heart beats
so rapidly, she can hardly count it. I saw her in one of these
attacks, and the pulse was between 141 and 150. She feels so
weak and ill then that she is unable to follow her occupation
which is that of a clerk; she is now living at home with her
parents. Poor, unfortunate girl, she had polio-myelitis as a
child, and her left leg is shortened and she walks with a bad
limp.

Prescription was: *Fraxinus americana* 1st centesimal, 5
drops night and morning, and *Veratrum album* 6 three times
a day for the dysmenorrhoea, while the pains were severe.

28.9.37. — Two months later. The periods have been up to
time, two periods since the first visit at four-weekly intervals,
the first time ever since she can remember! She still has
severe pains, but has taken nothing for it. On examination
uterus + + anteflexed, soft — above symphysis pubis, the
fibroid in the anterior wall is much smaller.

I looked her over again and noticed that she had many
warts on her chest and head, and brown moles here, there
and everywhere; she had never been vaccinated; but warts
and moles pointed to a latent sycotic infection, probably
dating back to grandparents. She was pale, her skin was dirty
whitish-grey, her hair was greasy and very dark, almost black.

(1) *Medorrhinum* 30, weekly doses.

(2) *Colocynth* 30, as required for the uterine pains. To
continue the *Fraxinus americana* 1st potency as an organ
remedy in between the periods.

16.11.37. — Periods regular, clots gone; all this since end
of July — pains still severe, relieved by *Colocynth*. Various
fears, fears of heights — fear of walking in the streets. *Argent.
nit.* 30.

Uterus much smaller; no sign of a fibroid now.

1.2.38. — Uterus small, anteflexed, fibroid cannot be
found.

Many nervous symptoms, has 'doorstep anxiety' — palpitations — anticipates trouble.

Causticum 6 three times a day prescribed mainly on the

history of the old poliomyelitis.

26.4.38. — Periods regular — has rheumatism of hip joints and knees and arms which is worse during cold, dry weather. Elimination is taking place, as is shown by muscular pains, the nervous symptoms and fears are much improved; the tachycardia is less troublesome. She is so much better that she is thinking of going back to work! Uterus is small, no return of fibroid so far. To continue *Fraxinus americana* mother tincture 5 drops night and morning, and *Veratrum album* 6 four-hourly for dysmenorrhoea.

I did not hear anything of this patient until the end of September, 1938, for five months in fact.

She had been so much better that the psychologist had advised her to try a job of work for a change and had referred her to a local panel doctor (she lived on the south coast).

She went to him for a cold and he was extremely rude to her for going up to London for psychological treatment, 'women doctors make too much fuss'. Examined her vaginally and was extremely scathing, as the uterus was normal and there was no fibroid. He did not believe there ever was a fibroid, he was the surgeon at the local cottage hospital and a fibroid could only be dealt with surgically and could not disappear with medicine. My patient assured him that a woman surgeon at one of the women's hospitals had diagnosed the fibroid and that another, a homoeopathic physician, had confirmed the diagnosis and claimed she could remove the fibroid with medicines, and if there was no fibroid now, it only proved that the homoeopathic medicines had cured it. He pooh-poohed it all, and upset the poor woman who, however, continued to believe that there was a fibroid in July, 1937, and by April, 1938, the fibroid had gone; therefore logically speaking, homoeopathy had done for her what was promised her. No operation had been necessary.

I examined her again in September of this year and found the uterus of normal size and no trace of fibroid.

She had various fears still, fear of water, fear of strong light, fear of doing things wrong, fear of being scolded. For these fears she was given *Stramonium* 200; and I have just heard that she is much more self-confident and suffers less from her nerves.

A most satisfactory case from a homoeopathic point of view. The diagnosis was originally made by a well-known gynaecological surgeon, and the subsequent disappearance of the tumour was confirmed by another surgeon.

I do not need convincing any more that homoeopathy *can* prevent *operations* and can even remove tumours; but the general public does, and so do the general run of physicians who have never seen what homoeopathy can do, *if* the right medicine is found.

This girl had psychological treatment for nearly three years, and there was very little change in her condition, her nervous state, her tachycardia, her sleeplessness, her inability to work, until she had homoeopathic treatment.

Two and a half years of psychological treatment by itself did very little for her; nine months of homoeopathic treatment added to the psycho-analysis produced healthy nerves as well; and the girl is now self-supporting again.

I do not say that homoeopathy alone would have cured the psychical discord; but it needed the simillimum to finish off the case and produce a cure. Homoeopathy requires time, it cannot cure overnight; here it took about nine months to cure a diseased uterus as well as a diseased mind and diseased nerves. As I am always saying, homoeopathy treats the individual, takes hold of him or her and alters the diseased states and builds up anew from the revitalized centre.

SURGICAL CASES CURED BY MEDICINE
The first duty of a physician is to heal the person who asks for help and according to the centuries old oath of Hippocrates he swears not to cut anybody, but to give way to those who are practitoners in this work. Alas, the number of surgeons have increased and the art of the physician has accordingly been forgotten. And yet a physician can cure and should cure people without having resource to the lancet and the knife. Years ago people were under the impression that

homoeopaths never cut people or in more elegant language operated on people.

I must confess to my grief and sorrow, that this is not the case any longer, and many operations are done in Homoeopathic Hospitals for conditions which used to be treated *and cured* by medicines only. Haemorrhoids, rectal fistulas among others, used to be treated by the indicated remedy and disappeared. You find many examples of this in the old homoeopathic books. And yet when I was a house surgeon, the operations for piles were as common in homoeopathic hospitals as in the orthodox ones. This was a great disappointment to me at the time. But I must say I do remember a case here and there which was saved from the surgeon's knife. One of these cases, I recall, was a case of trigeminal neuralgia, a neuralgia of the fifth cerebral nerve, which supplies the face, and causes a most violent pain along the course of the different branches of this nerve if it becomes diseased. A devastating pain which nothing can and will relieve ever. This particular woman had treatment for at least two years at several of the general and nerve hospitals. They had given her pain killing drugs; she had rubbed in various liniments, Menthol and Camphor, etc. on her face, she had injections of alcohol into the nerve. Nothing had helped. The only remedy that was open to her, according to a famous surgeon, as the last desperate chance between life and death, was to open up the skull and dig out the large nerve ganglion of the fifth nerve — the Gasserian ganglion. A very dangerous and a very lengthy operation. She shrank from the ordeal, and having heard of homoeopathy, she came to see whether she could be saved from this serious operation and also be cured of her agonizing facial neuralgia. She was a very patient woman, grumbled but little. She used to sit up day and night, rocking herself to and fro, supporting her face, gently groaning now and then with the agony of the pain. She was given some of the more usual homoeopathic nerve medicines, such as *Mag. phos.* and *Spigelia* in low potencies without the slightest effect. I think quite a dozen remedies were tried out on her, and yet there she was always in her corner, moaning and rocking, oh so gently, and yet the pitifulness thereof! — A keen young house physician just fresh from the teaching of Professor Kent was given the chance, before passing on the case to the surgeon, to work out the remedy.

Quite an hour was spent in eliciting the symptoms, another hour looking up the remedy. It worked out to *Sulphur* and without consulting the visiting physician who had given permission to the tyro in homoeopathy, a dose of *Sulphur* 10*m* was given in the morning. On the customary round with the night sister, this ward was visited, and to the astonishment of the young doctor, no Mrs. S. was seen sitting up in the corner. 'Had she been moved? Had she died suddenly? Had her heart given out from the constant pain?' The young medico's face blanched with anxiety and she tip-toed to the bed. But no, there was the patient, peacefully sleeping the sleep of the just. The next morning this patient was the first visit the house physician paid, to be told that the patient had slept all night, the first time for months and months and there had been no returns of the pain up to that time, the grateful woman said. The patient was jubilant, the relief was so sudden and so unexpected. She stayed in the hospital for another week or so to make sure that the cure held good. But there was no recurrence and the patient kept in touch with the hospital for several months, until she was lost sight of. As you may have guessed, I was the tyro, and it was my first case on whom I tried out my newly gained knowledge.

Yes, homoeopathy *does sometimes* cure like that, instantaneously, miraculously, if the patient gives the right symptoms and the right remedy is found. Many times, however, the cure is much slower and the patient may lose faith and almost lose hope, specially if kind friends and relatives urge him or her to try surgery and praise the wonderful things surgery can do. It needs constant encouragement on the part of the physician for patients not to give up the treatment. I remember such a case in a woman in the early forties who was suffering from a neuritis of the median nerve, which affected the right hand. She was first seen at the end of December, 1935. The history was that she had been moving heavy furniture some 10 weeks previously and somehow injured her wrist. The wrist began to swell, there was constant pain in the right arm, which woke her up at night. She had to keep the arm out at right angles to the body on an air pillow to get any relief. The wrist felt as if it was going to burst, and there was numbness of the fingers and stiffness.

I found that the median nerve was caught up in adhesions at the wrist, and this was the cause of the pain and numbness. Her doctor had advised a surgeon, and this surgeon at the hospital talked of dividing this nerve higher up nearer the shoulder. Nothing else would do, she was assured. I told her that it was extremely doubtful whether it would work. The other nerves would take six months or more before they would replace the divided nerve, and as she had to earn her living, what would she do in the interval? She agreed to try out what medicines could do. *Ledum* 30 in repeated doses was given for her local symptoms. Seen again on January 26th, 1936. Had been away for 2 weeks rest at the sea, as she thought she was run down. Still complains of numbness of right middle fingers; there is thickening of sheath across the wrist in front, which presses on the median nerve. She had been to another surgeon at the instigation of a friend who was sure that surgery was the 'only thing'. The opinion of this second surgeon was to leave well alone and continue with medical treatment. Wise man!

Further *Ledum* 30 was given every night to help the nightly pains. February 4th, 1936, numbness of fingers still the same, worse heat, worse beginning to move, worse in bed, right wrist less swollen, ultra-violet ray treatment given which made it worse, *Rhus tox.* 30 three times a day. She was then put on further ultra-violet ray and infra-red light treatment, which she had twice weekly for several months, with a moderate amount of relief.

June 6th, 1936, still numbness of her hand and fingers, especially middle finger, contraction of tendons of right hand on waking up in the mornings and after holding hand still as when travelling in vehicles, pain in right hand when holding anything. The contraction of the fingers appeared like a closing up of the fingers on the palm of the hand, similar to an early Dupuytren's Contraction. The tendons of the fingers were tense and tight and barely opened at all, except with a great effort. The palmar fascia — the sheath binding the muscles and tendons together in the palm of the hand — was tense and the tendons were standing out like whipcords. The annular ligament of the wrist was thickened and swollen. The neuritis was not quite so painful. It certainly looked as if the case was going from bad to worse. The light treatment was not doing much good either, except perhaps psychologically.

It was noticed that the patient was loquacious, voluble to a degree, that she felt the heat very much, and that her pains and numbness and tenseness of the fingers were always worse during the night or early morning and improved as the day went on. The three-legged stool again, on which to base a prescription. These symptoms meant *Lachesis*, and *Lachesis* 30 was given.

July 7th, 1936, she rang up, said she was very much better, the first time in six months that she acknowledged feeling better, her fingers and hand were straighter in the mornings. Continue *Lachesis* 30.

September 18th, 1936, much better until last week. *Lachesis* 30.

November 13th, 1936, stiffness of arm and hand worse during night, worse in bed, pain after sleep, pains go up the arms, cutting pains with numbness, pain after sleep. The local symptoms were covered by *Lachesis* and *Rhus tox.*; but the general constitutional symptoms were more *Lachesis* than *Rhus tox.*, such general symptoms as being loquacious and voluble, feeling the heat, worse during the night, hot flushes, flushed face, etc.; so once more she was given *Lachesis* 30.

December 5th, 1936, general improvement, but the local condition still troublesome, *Lachesis* 50m.

February 15th, 1937, numbness of third finger on waking, worse morning, pain better on motion, worse lying down, worse on beginning to move. The same condition was beginning to affect the left hand and left fingers as well.

Conditions going from right to left and the other symptoms mentioned just now meant *Lycopodium*, which is the complement to *Lachesis, Lycopodium* 30 now given. The tendency to contraction of the fingers had disappeared, the swelling of the wrist had gone long ago. The thickening of the palmar fascia had also disappeared.

April 1st, 1937, just a slight stiffness of the fingers and hands now after sitting still for a long time, such as after taking a long bus ride, improved by moving the fingers.

Rhus tox. 30 three times a day, prescribed – everything else had cleared up.

This finished the case. She has been seen once again for a totally different condition, a prepatellar bursitis, which cleared up quickly after *Ruta* 30 t.d.s. It took about fifteen months to cure this case of median nerve neuritis, followed by Dupuytren's Contraction of the palmar fascia. But the neuritis began to clear up and improve as soon as the general constitutional symptoms were made clear. It is difficult for the ordinary patient untrained in homoeopathic methods, to forget about the local pains and give correct symptoms of the real ego. Once the peculiar symptoms of each individual are made out, and the right constitutional medicine is given, the local condition will disappear with the improvement of the patient.

This woman was saved from a serious operation, the results of which were extremely problematical, and might have led to complete paralysis of the median nerve for months and perhaps forever. She has a perfectly useful hand, and shows no signs of neuritis or thickening or swelling of the various ligaments and tendons of the hand and fingers.

Lachesis in repeated doses was necessary, followed by its complement *Lycopodium*, to achieve this result.

This patient, I know, is extremely grateful *now* to have been spared this operation. She was able to follow her occupation the whole of the time she was having her treatment, which certainly would not have been possible if she had had an operation. It would have meant months of unemployment and much treatment, massage, electrical and ultra-violet ray treatment. It was very difficult at times to go against the advice of various interfering friends who were anxious to urge her to have the operation. One of these indeed was willing to pay for the operation! — but did not offer to pay for her medical treatment. Conservative treatment surely is better than the knife, and worth making an effort for.

This reminds me of another case of Dupuytren's Contraction I saw and treated some six years or more ago and saved from a crippling operation. Dupuytren's Contraction of the palm of the hand is rare in women, but this woman who was in the late forties, when I saw her, had helped her husband in his business which was flag making and rope making, and it meant letting the coil of the rope go through her left hand with the fingers slightly flexed on the palm, forming a tunnel. In order to keep her husband's business going while he was at the front from 1914-18, she did practically all the work and strained her fingers. The contraction of the fingers developed soon after and by the time I saw her, the little finger and ring finger of the left hand were bent over completely and could not be straightened at all. The middle finger was stiff and was beginning to be pulled over on to the palm, and the index finger was tending to follow suit. She had shown her hand to various doctors, and had desultory treatment off and on without it making any appreciable difference. She showed it to me more as a curiosity without expecting any help. She was a big, fat, blousy woman, with highly coloured cheeks, skin coarse and thick, inclined to be untidy and dirty and casual, felt the heat very much, had headaches on top of the head, sinking feelings of the abdomen about eleven o'clock in the morning. All *Sulphur* symptoms, so I gave her *Sulphur* 6 three times a day for a considerable period, on and off for nine months, with this result, unexpected by her — namely the fingers straightened completely, the tight fascia of the palm loosened and became normal, and there was free movement of all the fingers. She was duly impressed, and offered to go up to any Medical Society to show herself as a case of complete recovery from Dupuytren's Contraction, after she had been suffering from it for twelve years. Unfortunately the poor lady was too fond of her glass, she loved her drop of whisky, and was such a tippler that she developed diabetes and became totally blind from recurrent haemorrhages in the eye, so she had to be sent to a home for the blind. When I last heard of her, I was told that her hand was still quite normal and the contraction of the fingers had not recurred.

Poor thing, I could not persuade her to give up the drink; many times she was found maudlin by her neighbours. I could save her from an operation, but not from the consequences of too much whisky. The patient must co-operate with the physician and be strong minded enough not to give way to weakness. There is no specific medicine for Dupuytren's Contraction as such, but Dupuytren's Contraction of twelve years' duration in a *Sulphur* patient was cured without operation by doses of *Sulphur* in a few months, and early Dupuytren's Contraction, associated with neuritis of the median nerve, was cured completely by *Lachesis*, because the patient herself showed *Lachesis* symptoms. The next Dupuytren's Contraction I may see, may require a completely different medicine. In the same way the neuritis of the trigeminal nerve was not cured by a nerve medicine, but by the medicine required by the general characteristics of the patient in question.

Treat the patient, each man or woman, as an individual and do not treat the disease, the pathological entity as such; the vital force will be stimulated by the constitutional remedy, given on the sum total of the symptoms, and if there is enough reaction left, the pathological disease will be cured.

CHAPTER TWELVE

TUMOUR OF THE BREAST

A woman is always terribly distressed whenever she discovers a 'lump in her breast'. With all the cancer propaganda which has been going on for years, this is only natural; all the same one wishes that people would realize and remember that lumps in the breast can be cured by medicinal means, and that operations are *not* always essential. The usual procedure of course is to send the patient into hospital or nursing home and have the swelling removed, regardless whether it is malignant (cancer) or not. 'It might turn into cancer,' she is told; and the most dire results are predicted if she should not carry out the doctor's orders and go into hospital for an operation. I have watched a patient now for many months with such a condition and as far as I can tell at the present moment, she is cured.

She came to me at the end of October, 1937, with the history of the right breast being struck violently by a tennis ball two months previously. At the end of August, after the injury she went to the local doctor who did not think much of it; the bruise did not appear for two weeks. There was a large swelling the size of a tangerine orange above the nipple; the whole breast was badly discoloured, purplish-blue in colour, the nipple was retracted; there were no enlarged glands. On the history she was given *Arnica* 30, night and morning for a week.

11.11.37. Swelling slightly smaller, softer and not so blue. Repeat *Arnica.*

18.11.37. Swelling very tender. *Bellis perennis* 30, to be repeated nightly for a week.

25.11.37. Tenderness *gone* and discoloration gone – no difference in size.

9.12.37. Swelling softer, slightly smaller — very nervy, hot flushes, fortnightly periods. *Sulph.* 30.

16.12.37. No change in swelling of breast. *Bellis perennis*, 1st cent. potency. 14 powders, one to be taken every night.

20.1.38. Swelling much diminished in size. Continue *Bellis perennis*.

27.1.38. Felt poorly; both hands went dead in the afternoon, very nervy; feeling of tremulousness and shaking inwardly. *Ignatia* 30 night and morning.

3.2.38. Lump slightly softer. *Bellis perennis*.

I was wrong in giving *Bellis Perennis* at night. It produces nervous symptoms, disturbed nights and bad dreams; this would have been avoided if *Bellis* had been given in the day time.

17.2.38. No glands palpable. Repeat.

3.3.38. Lump not nearly so hard. *Phytolacca* 30 (1).

24.3.38. Only a tiny nodule now in the breast. *Phytolacca* 30 (1).

7.4.38. Repeat *Phytolacca*.

5.5.38. Has a severe cold, with herpes of upper lip. *Natrum mur.* 30 (1).

26.5.38. Breast worse again; left breast is enlarged and tender all over. Menstrual period very dark, almost black at times. Sleeps well, *Lach.* 30 (one dose).

2.6.38. Lump in breast larger. *Bellis perennis* ∮ t.d.s.

9.6.38. Complained she gets pain in her forehead twenty minutes after taking her medicine (the *Bellis*); could not sleep with her headache, feels light-headed — perhaps I was wrong. I should not have repeated the mother tincture of *Bellis* so often. The late Dr. Cooper found he got much better results in breast tumours, by giving one dose of the mother tincture and letting it act for some time. I had doubted this; but seeing the aggravation this woman suffered from the repeated doses, I made a note of it — for the future.

16.6.38. Period during last week; no clots, the colour is much improved.

23.6.38. No pain in her breast; is worried and nervy about her only child, very hysterical. *Ignatia* 30 night and morning.

7.7.38. Cannot keep legs still in bed, felt better the last few days. *Ignatia* 30 night and morning.

15.9.38. Not so nervous; still a small nodule felt in right breast; *Silicea* 30 ordered to absorb the last remnant of the swelling.

22.9.38. Periods regular, no trouble during period. Headache day before period; irritation all over the body, after going to bed, wakened up by the irritation. Bed-clothes are light, irritation not due to being too hot in bed; feels better in herself. Nodule hardly noticeable.

6.10.38. Much better in herself; irritable erythematous eruption all over, pimples on shoulder and back; feels heat — the *Silicea* is evidently acting as an eliminating agent and throwing out psoric manifestations. *Sulph.* 30.

27.10.38. Right breast well. Repeat *Sulph.*

3.11.38. A cold; sore throat, drawing pains at arm and hand, continual aching; also pharyngitis, sneezing, with a good deal of phlegm. Again psoric manifestations, and aggravations after the *Sulphur*. All the symptoms only manifested on the right side.

10.11.38. Everything was going on swimmingly until one day during the week, on trying to get on a crowded bus, she was pushed and received a heavy knock on her right breast, again a slight swelling showing; bruised at breast, pumping sensation in veins of right arm — glands of axilla nil. To wear a firm brassière for protection. *Arnica* 30 t.d.s.

17.11.38. Return of hard swelling in breast, alas! *Phytolacca* 30, night and morning.

24.11.38. Right breast a shocking sight, larger than it had ever been, deep blue and congested, *hard* swelling size of small orange fixed to skin, several hard, knotty glands along the border of right Pectoralis major in the axilla. Perspiration of the axilla profuse and offensive. This fresh knock had started up the old trouble which evidently had only been quiescent, with redoubled force, and this time the glands were infected as well. Was all our struggle against malignancy in vain? Had the enemy won after all? *Carcinosinum* 30 (1).

The patient was not seen for seven weeks, not *until*

January 12*th*, 1939, when she presented herself again. I had been most troubled about her in my mind; had she got so much worse, had she taken alarm and presented herself at a hospital where she would be severely ticked off for not having come along earlier, to have her breast removed? They would say hard things about me for having tried to treat her by medicinal means; and what about my reputation in that particular neighbourhood? She was a poor woman, it is true, and a dispensary patient; all the same she mattered to me, and I was sorry for the sake of homoeopathy that this should have happened. Thus ran my thoughts. Then to prove my fears wrong, she turned up smiling. She felt perfectly well; she had been busy and not able to come, as she lived a long way away.

Periods regular every three weeks, no complaints — lump in the right breast practically all gone; glands right axilla barely noticeable. Perspiration in axilla very strong. Wears a brassiere now for protection. *Carcinosinum* 30 (1).

19.1.39. Has been having pains on top of her head and at the back of her head. Could not bend down or stoop, without a good deal of giddiness. Evidently I repeated the *Carcinosinum* too soon after the first dose and this was an aggravation. Dr. Koch in Detroit, in the States, a great cancer man who has cured many cases of cancer, declares that giddiness (vertigo) is an early cancer symptom. Indeed, he considers it to be a premonitory symptom, a precancerous one. Is this therefore a return of old symptom which one should get according to homoeopathic principles?

2.2.39. Glands in axilla gone; swelling of right breast completely disappeared.

9.2.39. Feels very well except for pains in legs, a heavy feeling as if her legs were weighed with lead from the knees downwards; noticed it during the last week. Has been having chilblains on the toes of her right foot this winter during December and January.

All these symptoms are outward manifestations of elimination, following on the doses of *Carcinosinum* given, the tumour and glands have disappeared again, and the patient is feeling well. The swelling (tumour) of the breast, after a treatment lasting over sixteen months, has gone. If there had not been the second injury in November, she would have been well by then. Now she is protecting her breast, so that she will not be so liable to get it injured by a knock.

This has been a most instructive case to watch and taught me several things. If she had not been such a poor woman, I should have put her on a vegetarian diet and forbidden all meat and fish. But this is almost impossible to carry out in a poor home. If she had been able to follow a vegetarian diet, I could have got her well more quickly.

She still needs careful watching, but I am not afraid that she will leave me now. I have proved to her what homoeopathy can do. It is the people who get tired of the long treatment required in chronic constitutional diseases and leave you in the middle after only a short trial, who are so annoying and aggravating. Of course it is their loss; but the cause of homoeopathy suffers as well. For the homoeopathic remedies work slowly: they stimulate the vital centre and the actual repair of the damage done in the past takes time.

Why have an operation if homoeopathy can do as well, indeed, it usually does better. There is always the risk of disseminating the cancer cells all over the body through the blood stream during the course of an operation. True this does not always happen, but I have seen many cases die within a few months of the operation. If a patient survives five years after the complete removal of the breast, it is reckoned a complete cure. The late Dr. Burford had many cancer cures to his credit who survived longer than five years. And many other homoeopaths have done as well.

CHAPTER THIRTEEN

TWO CARDIAC CASES

In October, 1935, an old gentleman came tottering into my room, I was almost afraid he would die where he stood, and I did not think he was fit to be left to go about alone. He looked so feeble and frail. I put his age down at 78, and I was surprised when he told me he was just over 60. He had fallen into the hands of a so-called osteopath and naturopath, who had been starving him for several years on a diet which was only fit for rabbits; all green stuff, washed-out, watery cabbage and raw salads. He was underfed and suffering from hypervitaminosis, an overdose of vitamins and had been deprived for many months of the staff of life, the cereals. No bread was allowed him, only greens, salads, fish occasionally and fruit and a little milk. He used to be a hale and hearty man, weighing 11½ stones, his height being 5 ft. 10 in. Now his weight was down to 8 stones! He had lost 3½ stones in weight, and as I said, he looked so feeble, thin and emaciated he could hardly walk, was shaking and trembling where he stood, with bluish face, cyanosed lips, blue hands, skin dry and cold. He could not perspire at all, had a poor balance, the muscle sense was nearly gone, his feet felt numb, he could not feel the pavement when walking; he was so giddy, he had to hold on to the furniture and walked bent over a stick. His heat regulation centres were out of order too, he felt the cold terribly, felt hardly warm even sitting huddled up near the fire. Icy cold hands, icy cold back and legs and feet, suffered from chilblains, which were broken and discharging from the early autumn throughout the whole winter, and chilblains on his toes and feet and hands and even on his ears. It was a brisk autumn day and he was dressed up in layers and layers of clothes, woollen pants, two knitted woollen vests, scarves, great overcoat, and yet he felt cold and icy.

He suffered from a sinking sensation, as if he could fall down and sink through the floor, throbbing sensation of the neck, neuritis with shooting pains down the thighs — shortness of breath at night so that he could not lie down — indigestion, waterbrash, flatulence and distension of the abdomen after eating ever so little.

Very forgetful, suffering from anaemia of the brain, constipated of course; very serious, could not stand the slightest noise, self-centred, wanting to be alone, did not like company and disliked sympathy; heart feeble and irregular — pulse 60, slow; blood pressure low, only 100.

I put him on a full diet, he was to put on weight, eat two or three eggs a day, drink one to two pints of milk slowly through a straw, eat wholemeal bread, plenty of butter, cream-cheese, fish daily and meat three times a week, cream with fruit; bran and bran biscuits for his constipation. He was given *Lycopodium* 6, three times a day. I hardly expected to hear of him again, and thought he would die very shortly. I told him to go to bed as soon as he got home and stay there. As he came from the East coast I hardly expected him to turn up. However six weeks later he arrived again: he had been in bed for a fortnight and then started on the diet I had prescribed. He was a totally different man, had put on *nine pounds in weight* in a month, walked much better and was much stronger. Still some weakness in the legs, however, circulation still poor, but his chilblains were much improved, they had not broken so far. Ordered him to continue prunes and bran and hot milk for breakfast, which would regulate his bowels. To have a good mid-day dinner: cheese or egg dishes with two vegetables and fish every other day, meat twice a week, milky tea in the afternoon, with bran biscuits or wholemeal and bran cake; a supper similar to his dinner at 7 p.m. To go on putting on weight. *Lycopodium* 6, night and morning.

Early January, 1936. Reported much better, still easily startled by noises, gained 5 lb. in a month and nearly a stone in three months. To continue same medicine.

February, 1936. Not so shaky, circulation much improved,

slight chilblains on toes and left ear. Pulse steady, 84, blood pressure had gone up, was now 135. Heart sounds strong and regular. *Lycopodium* 30.

March, 1936. Still going well. Gained 1 st. 3 lb. since October, 1935. Complained of rheumatic pains in the left leg — had a nerve attack last week — otherwise much better.

April, 1936. Sleeping well, enjoying food, constipation much better, no indigestion, hands did not shake any more; standing now quite upright and straight, circulation much improved, no chilblains except slightly on the right ear.

He told me that two years ago he lost all his toe nails, and that the previous year all his finger nails dropped off as well. This year his nails had grown again and were quite normal. *Lycopodium* 30.

June, 1936. Rheumatism left shoulder, which was stiff and locked for several days — no nerve attacks now. Pulse steady and regular, 60 per minute. Blood pressure 135. His weight is now 9 st. 13 lb., he had gained almost two stones since the previous October.

September 3rd, 1936. Not quite so well, had an attack three weeks ago, fingers and toes went stiff and dead — felt sleepy all day. Weight still the same. *Lycopodium* 30.

November, 1936. Weight 10 st. 10 lb., in excellent health, no signs of chilblains.

I have not seen him since, but heard that he is hale and hearty, and no longer a feeble old man with one foot in the grave; after all he is not so very old, barely 63 years of age, and should enjoy many more years of life.

With a sensible diet, helped by the appropriate remedies, this gentleman with a feeble heart, poor circulation, low blood pressure was restored to health and strength.

In this case you can see how it follows again the rule that as a man returns to health, the symptoms leave him according to certain rules; from the more important internal organ they go to the more superficial tissues; from the liver and the heart to the muscles and the joints.

Now for another case, this time a lady.

In April, 1935, I heard from a doctor in the country that

he had seen Mrs. D., a patient of mine whom I had treated off and on for years, mainly for accidents in the past, who was suffering in his opinion from a failing heart, a serious myocarditis with degeneration of the heart muscle, high blood pressure, 200-210 mm., and albuminuria.

She was 75, feeble and unsteady and he considered she would not live very long. He had put her to bed, but she refused to stay in the country and was coming back to her town residence shortly. I saw her a week later and discovered, as the doctor had said, high blood pressure, an irregular pulse, every third beat intermitted, sometimes it would go very fast, then the rhythm altered and it became slow, then it stopped altogether for a beat or so. The heart was dilated; face bluish and congested, ankles swollen; a trace of albumen in the urine. She seemed very tired, collapsed and feeble; ordinarily she was most energetic and a strong-minded autocratic nature, would not be ruled by anybody, was a law unto herself. She allowed herself to be put to bed for a week and after that she was ordered not to get up until 11 a.m., after breakfast in bed, and she was told to rest on the couch in a covered verandah on the roof garden of her house. She spent three months like that, was very tired, collapsed and done up, specially the heart would play her up. I cut down her diet, she was used to a very rich diet: meat and meat soups twice daily, bacon and eggs and coffee for breakfast, milk puddings and cream, followed by a rich substantial lunch; cake and coffee after lunch and a four-course dinner with thick soup, fish, meat and suet pudding for dinner, followed again by coffee. She was very reluctant to cut out the meat and the coffee, she did not like tea, except good strong Darjeeling tea in the afternoon. She hardly touched vegetables, she did not like brown bread, but was very fond of rich cake, thick slices of Scotch fruit buns and pastries.

An extremely proud, reserved and silent nature, and very difficult to handle; would not admit that she felt ill. For her heart weakness and as a heart tonic she was given *Crataegus φ*, three drops three times daily, and for her sickness and collapse, *Sulphur* 6, night and morning. She made a very slow recovery, much too slow for her own impatient nature. For three months she led a very quiet life, just moving from bed to couch on the roofed-in verandah. The heart was getting stronger, the pulse-rhythm was getting more regular; but I knew that the *Sulphur* was not the absolute simillimum. I had given it for the weariness, the tiredness and the disinclination to move and exert herself. On examining the progress of the case frankly and without bias, I had to admit to myself that rest alone without the *Sulphur* would have done just as much good. I considered the *Crataegus* helped the heart; but the general condition was no different from what I had seen in heart cases with rest alone.

I continued to observe and watch and gradually a picture formed in my mind, helped by the observations of the confidential maid who had been with her for half a life time. I found she was extremely reserved and reticent, never talked about her own sorrows, but had been cut to the quick by the death of her only son and the sudden loss of her husband; she was estranged from several members of her family; hated sympathy which made her angry, very irritable specially in hot weather; the sudden collapse had come on after a great friend of hers had let her down and she was silently annoyed about it. She felt the heat very much, was very tired and exhausted in the mornings, had a great liking for salty food, for meat, for milk, for bread and for sweet things. Her skin was sallow, yellow, 'livery' and shiny; her eyes were yellowish. I saw at last, she must be *Natrum muriaticum* constitutionally, and eventually in September, when I had pieced it together, I gave her her constitutional remedy, the *Natrum mur.* 6, night and morning. The progress was almost startling after this. She became energetic, she went back to her committee meetings, her daily round of social engagements, and her visits in the parish. And after several weeks she suddenly admitted 'she felt so much better, but her skin was irritating intensely, what could she use for it, might she use some calamine to stop the irritation?' I found her arms up to her shoulders, her neck and back were covered with large patches of a macular eruption. I was most enthusiastic and pointed out that she was eliminating the toxin from the heart, that this was a dermatitis of gouty origin, and she was well on the way towards a cure. She was not convinced; but for my sake bore with it for several months. I continued the *Natrum mur.* first in the 6th potency and later in the 30th. The heart became regular, the dilatation disappeared, the blood pressure went down to 170 from 210, and she regained nearly all her old vigour. After all she was 76 and a year after the old country doctor had only given her a few weeks to live, she went about as of old. She would never acknowledge that her heart had given her trouble.

Three years later she was still alive and carrying on. It is never safe to predict a person's death, even old people have a way of pulling through, especially if homoeopathic medication is used.

Another example proving the correctness of the Law of the Direction of cure: that is from within outwards, from the more important vital organ to the less important, superficial one; from the heart to the skin. A physician who knows his Materia Medica will continually come across cases which show this sequence.

Blood pressure is made much of and is a bug-bear to many people. A diseased heart can be made to carry on with remedies, and there is no need for such so-called heart tonics as *Digitalis* and *Strophanthus*, and high blood pressure can be reduced sufficiently, so that a person can lead a useful life even though approaching the seventies. Homoeopathy has been known, if intelligently applied, to increase the expectation of life by many years.

CHAPTER FOURTEEN

BOILS AND CARBUNCLES

Boils, carbuncles and furuncles are different degrees of the same condition, a septic infection of the skin and the integuments with the staphylococcus; they are due to being 'run down', and are often associated with diabetes and kidney diseases. They are very painful, unsightly and have a disconcerting habit of appearing in consecutive crops. They belong to the borderland between surgery and medicine and the physician more or less successfully deals with it by ordering yeast internally or vaccines or injections with some preparation of manganese. Usually the treatment is a lengthy one, alas, under the orthodox methods.

One of the latest attempts of dealing with this troublesome complaint is by means of the modern cure-all and latest panacea for all septic or semi-septic infection; the famous Prontosil. A well-known dermatologist recently developed a boil in his nose with malaise and high temperature. He managed to subdue it and cure his boil within a few days with repeated doses of Prontosil, and he claimed this method as being superior to the usual method by vaccines. One swallow does not make a summer, and whether this preparation of sulphonamide would always work in the same manner, one does not know. Modern medicine only works by trials and precepts; there is no scientific foundation on which they can test their various treatments; so they are ever changing and altering. I have read lately several medical books which had been published at intervals of a decade, and each book recommended something different for boils!

I have seen many cases of boils and such like in my time, and like the famous dermatologist mentioned previously, I experienced them on my own self. At the end of the 1914-18 war, after the time of stress and strain and insufficient food and wrong food — such as lack of fat and the enforced use of fat made from clarified cocoa butter, I also developed carbuncles; at least three I can recall, which I treated surgically with foments and self-administered ethyl chloride local anaethesia, and incision of the septic focus, followed by the internal administration of *Hepar sulph.* and later *Silica* in isolated doses. I managed to clear up this condition in a little over a week, and there was no recurrence; so, judging from the record of our famous colleague, I did not do so badly with my unorthodox treatment. But still I suffered a great deal of pain, and in my own mind *Hepar sulph.* and *Silica* helped only moderately. Since then, in the last three years or so, I have discovered a method of dealing with carbuncles which is almost miraculous; it is like waving a wand, hey presto! and it is gone. And this not only in isolated instances; it very rarely fails, and then only if the symptoms do not correspond; in such cases, *Arsenic* or *Anthracinum* may be indicated.

The fame of this treatment has spread in various directions; I know a lady, for example, who has very little use for doctors and their medicines and less than no use for our method of minute doses; but she *does* believe in this treatment for boils and carbuncles, and wherever she can she recommends it and indeed there is now in her house a stock of this medicine, in case it should be wanted urgently.

I must tell you about two of her recent cases. On one of her shopping expeditions she noticed that the assistant behind the counter looked ill and that her face was disfigured with an enormous boil on her chin. She complained that she had had it for nearly a week and that her panel doctor could or would do nothing for it, and had just ordered some lotion for it, probably magnesium sulphate! My lady friend energetically enlarged on the wonders of the special pills she knew of, which cleared up boils very quickly, and the assistant, worn out with much pain and suffering, was only too willing to try anything, especially as her holiday was due the next week and she did want to enjoy it and not have to spend it repairing a damaged body. Unfortunately it was

Saturday midday and the remedy could not be procured until Monday, and by that time the carbuncle had at last opened by itself and was discharging; but a second one had developed in its vicinity, and she was dreading another week of pain, and the idea of an enjoyable holiday seemed farther away than ever. The pills were given to her, she was ordered to take them three times a day, and nothing more was heard from her for at least three weeks, that is until after her return from her holiday. She then joyfully reported that the first boil ceased discharging almost at once and that the second boil came to nought; it vanished without giving any further trouble, and her holiday worked out according to plan and the boil did not return during the time she was away. *And,* furthermore, there has not been any recurrence of boils up to date, which must be about a year now.

Quite a different tale compared with the following: A nurse I know well and meet often has been plagued with crops of boils and carbuncles all over her body for over a year; she is faithfully carrying out all the treatments ordered. At times she is so ill she has got to stay away from work, and then she crawls back more dead than alive. She has had courses of injections of various kinds, stock vaccines and auto-vaccines, manganese and iron injections, and still these plaguey things come back! She has attended hospital and private doctors; and that is all they can do for her. I do not know whether Prontosil has been tried out on her or not. She is still hoping that some day the boils will leave her. I cannot coax her away from her doctor and his nostrums, though I feel sometimes like saying to her, 'For goodness sake give it up and let me have a try.' But medical etiquette forbids.

Now another case of my good Samaritan lady friend, who works good by stealth. She went into a chemist's and heard that the nurse attending to one of the counters was very seedy with a carbuncle on the back of her neck, a huge thing, the size of a small plate. This nurse had a similar one six months previously, with crops of smaller ones round it, which had been most troublesome. She felt so ill that she thought she would have to go off duty. *Ma chère amie* immediately sang the praises of this wonder-worker among pills for this complaint and promised to get them for her. By the next day they were procured and nurse took a pill at 11 a.m. and then went off duty. I think it was a Saturday and the usual half holiday. As she felt so unwell she went to lie down, and then took another pill a little while later.

By 4 p.m. she woke up and to her surprise felt ever so much better, indeed so well that she got up and played tennis all the evening. By the next morning the carbuncle had disappeared without discharging, without any further bother. She could hardly believe her eyes, and she also has had no further trouble, and this is several months ago.

Both these girls are most enthusiastic about the rapid and painless way these pills work, and so grateful at being relieved so quickly.

Now for the *name* of this medicine, which should really be proclaimed from the house-tops; it is also a very good example of the truth of Homoeopathy. This remedy is obtained from the Cuban spider, the *Tarentula cubensis*, which lurks in the underground cellars and dark places and pounces upon its unsuspecting victim, the healthy, unconcious, experimental prover of the Hahnemannian lore. Find a healthy person and try out your medicine on him and notice his reactions, Hahnemann ordered; and from the reactions and symptoms you will get a picture of what a drug can do and can produce; and if you get similar symptoms in a sick person, you will be able to cure the disease by giving the similar remedy; such is his advice and on this is founded what we call homoeopathy.

Now this Cuban spider bites a person and this person develops promptly without fail in a few hours a boil on the place where he was bitten, which gets worse and worse and may spread and last for weeks and may even kill weakly children through septic absorption. Here is the septic boil developing after a bite; Hahnemann says 'like cures like'; therefore, if you get a person who has boils or a carbuncle, or a crop of them, give him some doses of this spider poison or spider virus, and if the law is correct, this spider virus, the

Tarentula cubensis, will cure it. The bite of the spider produces objective symptoms, the boil — and it also removes rapidly and painlessly the objective, the visible sign of the disease, the boil in the sick individual not only now and then, not only occasionally, but in nearly every case. I have had many cases of cure and so have other doctors who have tried it. It is something which cannot be explained away.

You need not believe in Homoeopathy; it is not a faith cure; the two people I mentioned above did not know what they were given; they had no particular belief in it, they were cured in spite of themselves! Yes, I always maintain that *Tarentula cubensis* given in exceedingly small doses is an object lesson, and a proof of the truth of Homoeopathy. Like cures like. The spider's bite is followed by a boil, and the boil in another individual is cured by the spider in the minutest dosage, the 6th potency, 12th potency, or the potency I myself usually give, the 30th given for a few days, until the boil has gone.

Anthracinum in a high or medium potency may be necessary sometimes for the very large carbuncles with an extension area of hardened and oedematous tissues around, with swelling of the glands and with intolerable burning and a bluish-blackish discolouration. I have seen one or two cases like this, in which *Tarentula* proved to be ineffective and *Anthr.* cleared up this threatening and spreading condition in a few days.

If you want to convince anybody that medicines given according to homoeopathic principles work, give *Tarentula cubensis* for *boils*. It leaves no bad after effects; the boils do not recur and the patient feels well. What more can you possibly want? It is almost too simple; but seeing is believing, or should be. Alas! that so many should be so blind!

CHAPTER FIFTEEN

REMEDIES OF FEAR AND STRESS

During World War II almost overnight everything had altered, old values had gone, new ones had appeared. We had to accommodate ourselves to a totally different world, and one thing among others we had been told was to keep calm and collected. This is a difficult thing to do, when everything around one crashes; business and trade nearly gone. Many people who had responsibilities found themsevles reduced almost to the point of penury. Others found their family circle broken up, fathers separated from wives and children — not because they had been called up to face the enemy on the battlefield, but because the whole of England was now a potential battlefield and the weaker vessels, old and frail people, the children and their mothers had been moved out to presumably safer areas. This brought forth many new problems, problems of adaptation. Another problem we had all got to face was the problem of air raids, and A.R.P., as it is called in the short, snappy way, does not only mean splinter proof and blast proof shelters, sandbags and the rest, it also means putting on a mental armour to protect ourselves against the insidious enemy of fear and anxiety. Here Homoeopathy is a valuable friend and helps against the effects of fear which produce an empty feeling round the umbilicus, a burning, gnawing sensation, a cleaving of the tongue to the roof of the mouth, a shaking and trembling of limbs; all of it due to upset of the suprarenal gland.

There are several remedies in our pharmacopoeia which give us moral protection.

I mention the most common. There is *Argentum nitricum*, the fidgety, nervous individual whose nerves are all to pieces. He is always in a hurry, anxious hurry, so hurried and scared, he feels he must run or walk quickly, he can never walk fast enough, he feels he must fly, feels as if all the 'furies of the underworld' were after him, and he runs and runs until he is dead beat, always anticipates the worst, lives in a perfect welter of fear and anticipation, breaks out in a sweat at the mere thought of a raid. But this anxiety and fear brings on internal troubles and disturbances of the gastro-intestinal tract, the stomach refuses to digest anything, vomiting may come on quite suddenly when an air raid warning is sounded, or even diarrhoea set in. The stomach is full of gas and quantities of wind pass upwards which usually relieves the distension. Silver nitrate in the 3rd or 6th centesimal potency would relieve such an over-anxious, frightened, hurried individual, so that he can face the inevitable with more equanimity.

A remedy with very similar effects is *Gelsemium*. He is also in a state of funk due to anticipation, fear, shock from fear, sudden fearful surprises. As Kent puts it: A soldier going into battle gets diarrhoea. He becomes weak and exhausted and faint, and tired in all his limbs from sudden fear, from sudden shock, such as being awakened at night by a raid warning. Palpitations of the heart accompany this sudden shock. He has no courage, his limbs tremble; but he is struck dumb, almost paralysed with fear; the restlessness and hurry and anxious running about of the *Argentum nit.* patient is absent. Thus you have to individualize and find the right remedy for each state of nerves.

Another anxious, restless patient may want *Arsenicum*. Here you get great fear, great anxiety, great restlessness and prostration. Some people take the blackest view of any situation which might arise. These are the folk which will say, 'What is the use of doing anything?' They will wring their hands and wail: 'Where can I go? I am not safe anywhere; if I remain here, the bombs will drop here, and if I go away into the country, they are sure to follow me there.' These over-anxious people, who are much worse when alone, will need *Arsenic*, and it will calm the troubled waters of their mental fear and unrest.

Aconite also has many symptoms of fear. He is frightened

in a crowd, will not mix with people, afraid of public places and public shelters; full of anguish, full of restlessness, afraid of the dark, much affected by the black-out, dark streets, darkened rooms. He gets violent palpitations of the heart; fear attacks the heart, not stomach, and the umbilicus as *Argentum nit.* and *Gelsemium* do. He predicts the next bomb will hit him, and predicts the time of death. He broods over this, and this fear makes him sleepless, restless and full of anxiety.

We have another valuable remedy for fear in *Ignatia.* This is the hysterical individual who faints at the slightest provocation, collapses into the arms of the nearest male for protection; is tearful, nervous, full of twitches and jerks, full of grief; her husband is away, she is always sighing, she has a feeling of emptiness in the stomach and abdomen, along with trembling, is continually sighing, sad at having said good-bye to her son, or fiancé or her husband. She is apprehensive all the time that something may happen. *Ignatia* is the best antidote I know for the stressed feeling one gets after a sudden bereavement, when the unfortunate person who is left behind to face the world lies there with dry, burning eyes, hour after hour, and can hardly believe that it is true that her dear one has left her.

Do not forget either to have *Arnica* near at hand; it works wonders in injuries, falls, concussion, blast and so on, even fractures, dislocations are helped by it.

An A.R.P. worker came to the centre to have his elbow treated. Two days previously he was thrown by the blast from a high explosive bomb and his left arm and elbow were almost paralysed and numb. *Arnica* applied externally and *Arnica* 30, four hourly removed the stiffness and disability and pain in a few hours. Two days later, he could move his arm freely and exclaimed at the rapidity of the cure and sent several of his mates over for similar treatment.

For strained muscles after lifting heavy weights, etc., remember *Rhus tox.* 30, dissolved in water and taken as required four hourly until stiffness and pain clears up; you will not regret it.

For abrasions and wounds which are usually covered thickly with debris and dust from brick-dust of the blasted houses, and are apt to go septic at once, remember *Calendula* dressings applied externally; use *Calendula*, mother tincture, 15 drops to a wineglass of boiled water. This will cleanse the abraded surface and prevent sepsis. *Calendula* 6 given three to four times daily by the mouth will assist the healing process.

If sepsis has already set in, use *Hypericum*, mother tincture in the same strength and give *Hypericum* 6, four hourly. You will be surprised how quickly either one or the other of the above will heal the torn flesh. Do not waste your time applying iodine; bathing with *Calendula* and an external *Calendula* application or *Hypericum* does much better than boracic dressings or fomentations.

For septic eyes and eyes covered with grit, I also find *Calendula* lotion of the greatest use.

For burns, however extreme they are, I should use *Urtica urens*, mother tincture, for an external application, being careful to leave the dressing on for days, and if necessary, only moistening it, whenever dry, with the *Urtica Urens*. Give *Causticum* 6, internally, every 15-30 minutes at first for the pain and shock accompanying a burn. For deep burns, use the *Calendula* lotion instead of the *Urtica urens*. It is really astonishing how quickly the pain disappears and how rapidly the burn heals without scarring.

The nurses at the centre are most enthusiastic at the good results they get with this treatment, and to be quite frank, so am I. I never had such rapidly healing wounds in the old days when I used antiseptic dressings. It needs some courage at first to strike out for yourself and to do things contrary to the accepted teaching; but it is well worth while when you see the results.

Air raids are a thing of the past for the moment, but we have still nervous, fearful people around us, and their nervous symptoms will be relieved by the remedies mentioned, whatever *their* cause may be, provided the symptoms correspond.

Publisher's Note

There are still many places in the world today where war and internal strife are part of the present way of life. We see increasing violence in crime and in the powers of evil stirred up by the lower passions in man. Fears and emotions run riot and violent death marks each day for many people. So it is well we are still able, as always, to turn to Homoeopathy and find remedies of comfort and healing for the body and mind.

CHAPTER SIXTEEN

A CASE OF SEVERE EYE AFFECTION

Medicine is, or should be, the divine art of 'healing', and in the oath of Hippocrates, the wise Greek physician, who lived hundreds of years before Christ, a doctor swears that he will use that regimen which according to his ability and judgment, shall be for the welfare of the sick. 'The sick', mind you, not for the welfare of the drug houses and for the good of the pockets of the vested interests of the serum and vaccine manufacturers, who seem to run nearly the whole medical profession, except the few who see further than the rest and, full of divine discontent, dissociate themselves and search for truth wherever it may be found, this truth which is hidden in the deep well of Hahnemann's often cryptic writings and the many books left by his earlier pupils.

And what joy there is if one pearl of truth and wisdom after another is found in these old dusty books, truths which help one to heal, truly heal, precious human bodies and souls who are burdened not only with original sin but also burdened with the sins of their ancestors.

Such chronic diseases are difficult to cure right from the bottom, it is easy enough to suppress, to hide, to cover up the external manifestations of disease, by the modern methods of treatment; but the original disease is still there, and will break out again and again in a different place; and neither the person afflicted nor the treating physician or physicians will and can see the connecting thread.

I saw such a child afflicted with a deep-seated chronic disease, and have been able to follow her progress for the last six years. She came first at the age of six in May, 1934, for dermatitis after orthodox treatment for scabies, just having recovered from measles as well.

A miserable, pallid, thin, stoop-shouldered girlie, very

nervous and timid, crying easily at the slightest thing, literally hanging on to her mother's skirts, a mouth breather with enlarged septic tonsils and with septic teeth; also left conjunctivitis. *Sulphur* 30 given for the after effects of measles and suppressive treatment of scabies. She attended regularly and various remedies were given, *Pulsatilla* for her weeping, then later she was put on *Baryta carb.* 30 for about six months, as she was so timid and frightened of strangers. She improved on this, appetite was better and she was not so nervous and scared. Her tonsils did not improve and there was also some deafness and a great deal of pressure from the school authorities, who wished to have an operation for removal of the tonsils.

Gradually I noticed that the eyes were getting worse; there was a good deal of photophobia, and lacrimation from the eyes, so I sent her up to the local Eye hospital for further investigation. There it was found that the pupils would not dilate properly owing to deep-seated adhesions, which bound the iris to the posterior wall of the eye.

This diagnosis of the eye surgeon was an excellent pointer to the underlying chronic disease and the child was immediately put on *Lueticum* 30, though the Hospital was very urgent as well about the septic tonsils. She improved on repeated doses of *Lueticum* 30 at weekly and sometimes fortnightly intervals, and I noticed that the weeping from the eyes, the lacrimation, was less troublesome.

I do not approve of indiscriminate tonsil operations; but once the local school authorities are on the war path, it is almost impossible to refuse an operation. So the child was sent up to the throat department of a children's hospital on at least two different occasions. The first time she stayed in for nearly five days and was continually sick, a nervous type of vomiting, as the child was frightened of hospitals and operations. So they let her go. A second time she was admitted and this time she promptly developed bronchitis and again she escaped.

She improved in her general health, though she still could not see as she had ulcers on the cornea and photophobia, dread of light, and constant weeping whenever she turned her eyes in the direction of light. I asked for dark glasses from the eye hospital, but I got no co-operation, all they wanted was to 'operate on the tonsils'.

While the child was still so nervous, it was impossible to insist on this. In September 1935, she developed severe whooping cough and was under a local doctor for several weeks with a high temperature and presumably bronchitis. On October 3rd, 1935, she came back to the dispensary barely able to crawl, still whooping after six weeks of home treatment with nightly temperatures of 100 degrees. *Drosera* 30 given. She picked up well after *Drosera*, which was repeated on October 27th and again on December 12th and January 9th, 1936.

On January 30th, 1936, at last on the third attempt, she managed to stay the course and had her tonsils removed in hospital. This was followed by acute pharyngitis and inflammation of the throat, and the lacrimation from her eyes was very troublesome and the sight worse than ever. The operation evidently let loose some microbes hidden in the crypts of the tonsils! She was then sent by the school doctor to an eye specialist who very brightly suggested a blood examination, and ordered removal to a well-known eye hospital in the country for a course of anti-syphilitic treatment. Fortunately for the child's sake, this doctor did not have the knack of making himself pleasant to hospital patients, and continually put their backs up by his peremptory manners, so the parents refused point blank to give their permission.

Now the chase was fully on; the pack of hounds from the school authorities followed the sport and barked and bit at the parents for daring to contradict the verdict of the pundit at the hospital. The onus was on me, and so I sent her to the eye department of the Homoeopathic Hospital, where at last they prescribed dark glasses, so that the child could walk out in the streets without continually weeping.

On May 21st, 1936, she was put on *Hep. sulph.* 30 for the following reasons: syphilitic history, catches colds easily from the cold north-east winds, and is very cheeky at home. You see the homoeopathic treatment for two years had changed her nervous and retiring temperament!

She was kept on occasional doses of *Hep. sulph.* 30 until September, 1936, when she presented herself with a right-sided swollen knee, pain and tenderness behind knee and stiffness, and also some heat and redness. She was ordered rest in bed and given *Drosera* 30, which arrested the acute inflammation in the knee joint.

On October 8th, 1936, the right knee was found to be one-third of an inch larger than the left knee, but she was much better in herself and she had gained 11 lb. in sixteen months.

On January 14th, 1937, the right knee was still stiff and swollen. *Drosera* 30. Unfortunately she was then seen again by a visiting doctor at the school for the physically handicapped where she had been attending for a year, and this physician started another trail of trouble by ordering her to yet another general hospital for further syphilitic treatment. I sent her again to the Homoeopathic Hospital for an X-ray of the knee joint, where no bony abnormalities were discovered. *Silica* 30 was prescribed and the stiffness, etc., improved.

May, 1937, seen again by the eye surgeon at the Homoeopathic Hospital, who suggested further doses of the syphilitic nosode.

June 3rd, 1937, painless right knee, still swollen, however, ½ inch larger than left. 'Throws off her colds more easily than she used to.' *Tuberculin.* 30.

June 17th, 1937, profuse brown moles all over body — the sycotic element coming uppermost, thrown out by the action of the *Tuberculinum. Thuja* 30 ordered, which was followed by some nasal catarrh.

July 16th, 1937, still looks very pale, sleeps on her face, a further manifestation of the sycotic element. *Medorrhinum* 30.

September 2nd, 1937, no lacrimation from the eyes — no swelling of the right knee, *but* swelling and *pain of the right ankle.* She could not fasten her right shoe, right foot hot and swollen.

September 16th, 1937, stiffness right ankle and foot, worse on beginning to move. *Rhus tox.* 30 t.d.s.

September 30th, ankle less swollen, no pain. Continue *Rhus tox.*

October 7th, right ankle ¾ inch larger than left ankle. Eyes better, can stand light better, no lacrimation when facing light. Afraid of school, lessons worry her. *Lycopodium* 30 ordered.

November 4th, 1937, no pains in leg, but still walks stiffly. Very lively, does not like strangers, takes more interest in things. *Lycopodium* 30.

November 25th, 1937. Again seen by another so-called specialist at school who diagnosed rheumatism, and considered she had a healed heart lesion (not knowing anything of the previous findings of a positive Wassermann test and history of corneal ulcers and adhesions of the iris!). Once again I prevented her from being sent up to yet another hospital for further treatment for rheumatism!!

December 12th, 1937, very pale still, gained 18 lb. in two and a half years, very good result of treatment. *Bacill. sycotic.* 30.

February 10th, 1938, much better in herself, pains in stomach after onions. *Thuja* 30. Again followed by a running cold, sneezing, profuse discharge from nose.

March 10th, 1938. Mother volunteers the remark that eyes were first noticed to be bad after measles in 1934; on looking up back record this was found to be correct. As she had tendency to diarrhoea after fat food and onions, she was given *Pulsatilla* 30.

March 31st, 1938. Great improvement, no more diarrhoea after fat or after onions. Knee not stiff, ankle not swollen any more; gets on well at school now, is fifth in her class.

July 21st, 1938. No stiffness of knee or ankle for weeks, no gain in weight since April, 1938, extremely pallid still. *B. sycotic.* 30.

September 1st, 1938. 'The best August for four years.'

Eyes improving, right knee and right foot give no trouble. Gained 9 lb. in a year. *B. sycotic.* 30. Sent away from London to Dymchurch by school authorities 'for fear of war breaking out' and returned home on October 6th. After a month away, has lost 2 lb., is still very nervous, hates being separated from her parents and home. *B. sycotic.* 30.

October 13th, 1938, gained 2½ lb. after being back at home for a week; this shows how she reacted to her surroundings, and what a homebird she was. Kept under the action of *B. sycotic.* for several months with general improvement all round.

February 16th, 1939. Gained 11½ lb. in a year, big sturdy child, eyes not so much trouble, can sit and read books now fairly comfortably.

April 27th, 1939. Vision greatly improved. When she first went to school, could not even see the top row of the Snellen's Reading Cards, can now see the letters on the third row from the top.

June 22nd, 1939. No trouble with right knee or right foot, vision improving still more, also gaining in weight. *B. sycotic.* 30.

July 27th, 1939. Gained nearly a stone in a year, eyes much better, no photophobia, no lacrimation; still opacities on cornea round pupils. *B. sycotic.* 30.

Then the war broke out and she was not seen again until January 11th, 1940. No swelling of either right knee or right foot, vision steadily improving. Weight now 5 st. 10 lb. 12 oz., a very good weight for a child who is 11 years and 6 months old. She weighed only 3 st. 8 oz. in May, 1935, five years previously, and had thus gained 2 st. and 10¼ lb. in 4 years 9 months, a very good record. Went to an ordinary school and was doing well.

May 2nd, 1940. Seen by eye surgeon who was well satisfied; vision good, general health good, still some opacities on the cornea. Weight now 5 st. 12¾ lb. At last after five years of attendance, an interesting piece of family history was discovered. The maternal grandfather died after a fall and the mother let out in the course of conversation that he had been suffering from locomotor ataxia for many, many years. Here was the link that I had been looking for for years, the beginning of the syphilitic infection. The result was the unfortunate grandchild had been suffering from congenital syphilis ever since birth, almost complete blindness and general marasmus, until she was taken in hand and treated homoeopathically. No strong allopathic drugging was necessary, and only minutest doses of the appropriate remedies were given, and yet the blindness cleared up considerably, though she will never have 100 per cent vision. Did you notice, too, how the truth of the homoeopathic law was brought out during the course of treatment, which extended over several years? The homoeopathic cure of a deep-seated infection goes from above downwards, from within outwards — the law states. The serious deep-seated infection of the important internal organs, the eyes — was followed in due course by swelling and inflammation of the less important organs, the right knee joint. Then a little while later, the right ankle joint became affected, while all the time the sight and the general health improved, the psychological characteristics also improved, nervous instability went, the brain power, the power to learn and to retain facts improved. This is how it should be. A triumph for Homoeopathy. Even quite good homoeopaths shy at the homoeopathic treatment for syphilis, and think that this should be treated by orthodox methods, by arsenic or bismuth salts and whatever may be the latest orthodox way.

This case proves that this is unnecessary, that Homoeopathy can and does cure even such a deep-seated disease as syphilis, and that it cures without giving great discomfort to the patient. No need for painful intravenous injections of noxious drugs.

A further development occurred recently. Early June, 1940, this girl developed what was called by the school doctor impetigo of the left side of the face and forehead. This spread rapidly and when I saw it, the whole left side of the face, chin and nose was covered. I considered it was due to ringworm, a malignant, rapidly spreading type, which was traced to a badly infected cat living in the house. The ringworm was treated locally for two weeks without any effect. Then I remembered that Dr. Burnett recommended *Bacillinum*. I had no *Bacillinum*, but I gave her *Tuberculinum* 30, one dose, with appreciable difference to the ringworm in a week. Then I gave daily doses of *Tuberculinum* 30 for a week, and several days later the face was clear, not a vestige of ringworm! The child can read ordinary small print without glasses now and her general good health and progress is maintained.

Oh, that the day would dawn when Homoeopathy is taught properly in the medical schools. How much suffering, how much chronic ill health could be saved.

CHAPTER SEVENTEEN

HOMOEOPATHY IN SKIN DISEASES

On June 18th, 1935, a working class woman brought her boy aged 7 to the dispensary with mild impetigo of the face. In the background stood a much older girl, whose face was made hideous by being plastered thickly with an objectionable black ointment. I had asked whether she had been brought for treatment as well, to which the mother replied that she was attending a well-known skin hospital. Then the floodgates opened, the big girl began to shed tears and the mother joined in.

After a decent interval while they composed themselves, I heard that this skin trouble had first shown itself when she was five months old and had not abated since. In fact during the thirteen years which had passed by, she had attended all the hospitals in the neighbourhood, she had tried three large teaching hospitals, she had been to two special skin hospitals, she had had sunlight treatment, had been away several times for convalescence for months at a stretch at sea-side homes, and only last week the specialist at the skin hospital had shrugged his shoulders and said that she would have this skin trouble all her life, nothing more could be done for her, she would always require treatment, and must always use some ointment. One wonders what for? It did not cure or even remove the skin eruptions and it certainly could not be said to add to her appearance, as this black tar ointment, unpleasant to look at and with an unpleasant odour, had to be applied thickly round the lips and back of the ears.

The child was at an age when she began to take notice of her own appearance and wanted to look her best and disliked being teased by her school friends about the disfigurement of her face. Somewhat rashly perhaps I offered to cure the child, provided she was kept under treatment for a sufficient length of time. The mother would hardly believe that the girl could ever get rid of her 'skin trouble', but was willing to give the treatment a trial.

The girl was thick set and stoutish, with a pale, pasty complexion, a heaped crusty scabby eruption round the mouth and a similar scabby eruption in the bends of the elbows and at the back of both knees, with bleeding cracks. A typical *Graphites* rash, so on June 20th, 1935, *Graphites* 30 was given and all local treatment was forbidden. Seen on June 27th, the remark was made that the cracks of the skin did not bleed any more and that the irritation was much worse at night, due to this.

July 4th, elbows clearing, left knee healed — face completely clear, has not had a clear skin since November of the year before.

July 11th, lips cracked. *Graph.* 30, one dose.

September 5th. Skin improving since July; no thickening of skin. Mother says, she has never had such a good time.

September 19th. Return of skin trouble on face. Child is going in for a scholarship.

October 24th. Face clear.

All through the winter until the end of March, 1936, the skin all over the body remained clear, there were no bleeding cracks, as in the past; then the skin round the lips began to thicken again and swell up, so another dose of *Graphites* 30 was given.

On May 21st, 1936, she had a sharp attack of chicken pox, for which she was given *Ant. tart.* 30, night and morning, and which cleared up the spots in under a week.

June 25th. Slight return of dermatitis on flexures of both forearms and knees, and very slightly on face. *Graph.* 30, three doses, one nightly on three consecutive nights.

July 9th. Skin rather worse, probably due to reaction after the *Graphites*, however, by July 23rd the face and knees were once more clear; September 3rd, 1936. Very tired, lies about all day. After a stay at the sea-side and exposure to the sun and salt spray, eyelids were swollen and red and the elbows, knees red, scurfy and cracked — *Graphites* 1,000th potency.

September 12th, 1936. Much better, not so tired, eyes not

swollen.

September 17th, 1936. Not so tired, not lying about any more. Skin better, feels happier as she does not look such a sight. No further treatment required until May 27th, 1937, well over eight months later, when there was a slight cracking round the mouth. Though the child was nearly sixteen years of age, no periods yet. On June 25th, three nightly doses of *Graphites* 30 were given. The period came on for the first time at the end of June. (A *Graphites* patient has usually delayed and scanty periods — a further proof of the correctness of the remedy in this particular girl.)

September 9th, 1937. Return of skin trouble, very distressed and weepy because of the appearance of her face. No period since the end of June. Feels cold and miserable and depressed. *Graphites* 30 (three doses), followed by rapid improvement. Another period came on at the beginning of November, and after that the periods appeared regularly every three weeks without any pain or discomfort.

March 9th, 1938. Face well, skin soft and smooth all over body.

June 16th, 1938. Skin round mouth cracked and chafed. No M.P. since February. *Graphites* 30.

September 8th, 1938. Skin round mouth thickened and bleeding. *Graphites* 30. No real 'breaking out' on skin for the last twelve months. The period showed itself again within a week of medicine.

October 29th, 1938. Irritating eruptions at bends of elbows due to wearing a woollen jumper. 'Three years since she had a bad arm.' *Graphites* 30 (three doses).

November 3rd, 1938. Arm worse, lips swollen and split, very upset and worried about it. *Graphites* 30 (three doses).

March 2nd, 1939. Slight roughness on face and cracking after using a theatrical make-up. *Graphites* 30.

July 13th, 1939. No trouble with periods. Some patches of skin trouble on the elbows. *Graphites* 30 (three doses in 24 hours).

Since that date ten months ago the skin has remained quite clear and smooth and this young girl has remained well and happy.

What she has been saved! No local treatment, no horrible disfiguring salves and ointments for five years, only a few occasional doses of homoeopathic medicine. She is now nearly nineteen years of age and busy and happy at her job.

Skin diseases are to the average person loathsome, and how unpleasant the usual treatment is, and how much more pleasant our way of tackling this job is. Skin diseases are due to something wrong inside the body, due to metabolic errors, the soil is wrong; therefore skin eruptions should not be treated by applying lotions or ointments or pastes, which would only suppress the actual trouble and drive it under-ground, there to cause further and more serious interference with the normal functions of the cells. This is said to be an antiquated idea according to some doctors; but one has proved the truth of this statement so many times to one's own satisfaction that in spite of the opinions of distinguished doctors I repeat it. Skin troubles, skin eruptions, should be treated from within by suitable medicines. It can be done; it may take a long time; and it is always worth while to make the attempt. Now don't run away with the idea that *Graphites* is always necessary to cure skin troubles. You may need any one medicine, according to the nature and character of the eruptions, the reactions of the skin to temperatures, to water; whether there is any bleeding, any discharge; whether there is any itching, any irritation. And it is frequently most difficult to find the right medicine.

Impetigo of the face is a common occurrence among the school population in the poorer quarters of the cities and villages, and it takes weeks sometimes to cure it, as I know to my cost after years of experience at a dispensary.

I find that *Antimonium tart.* in the 6th potency, or even higher in the 30th potency, without any local applications – except powdering with some starch powder, will clear up the crusts and sores rapidly. Do not attempt to remove the crusts, leave them dry and exposed to the air without any dressings, and many times I have managed to clear and remove the impetigo within a week and certainly under a fortnight. One does see some very bad cases where the impetigo has spread all over the face and ears. I find *Antimonium tart.* much better for impetigo than *Sulphur.* And that reminds me, *Sulphur* ointment should not be applied to skin eruptions ever; it produces an eruption of its own, and is therefore homoeopathic or similar to many skin diseases.

This recalls the cure of another skin case of several years' standing. A lady developed dhobi rash, a disease of the tropics, and for well over 2½ years had an eruption all over the palms of both hands, for which she had prolonged treatment at a London hospital, mainly by ultra-violet rays. This suppressed or removed the eruption on the hands and brought out nasty crops of boils. So it went on, boils alternating with the eruption on the palms. The skin burnt and there were deep bleeding cracks on both hands, a badly disfigured nail of the right index finger — this finger was continually shedding its nail, as well as an irritation and burning of the groins. Also scaling and itching at the back of the ears. *Petroleum* 30 given. No local treatment advised except olive oil.

A week later there were deep cracks on the hand and much itching at night in bed. Rheumatism of the left ankle. *Sulph.* 30 ordered.

The following week, slight improvement of the hands, itching slightly more bearable at night. *Sulph.* 30.

Two weeks later a boil developed on right shoulder, which cleared up after half a dozen doses of *Tarantula cubensis* 30, without opening or discharging.

A week after this, acute rheumatism and stiffness and pains of both legs and ankles; has to walk with a stick. *Rhus tox.* 6 alternately with *Bryonia* 30, four hourly, ordered.

A month later, when seen, the palms of hands were clear and had been for nearly three weeks, and the rheumatism had also disappeared.

A skin eruption which had lasted for 2½ years in spite of expert treatment, or because of it?— was cured from within by a few doses of the appropriate medicines, in six weeks!!

This happened nine months ago and there has been no recurrence so far, even the nail on the index finger has remained sound. Indeed, my patient was most alarmed when the acute rheumatism appeared and talked of going to Spa treatment at Buxton or Droitwich, I cannot recall which now; but there was no need even for that, *Rhus tox.* and *Bryonia* took care of it and Homoeopathy had conquered again. She had also asked for a pathological examination of the eruption on the hands, but before this could be carried out, the rash had disappeared! So I do not know whether it was the result of the tropical disease or not, or what the diagnosis really was. The result was satisfactory both to the patient and to me, that is all that matters, do you not think so?

Is not our method of treating 'skins', as the medical student calls it, much more attractive than messy local applications? And are not the results gratifying as well? Would it not revolutionize the orthodox treatment if they would allow us to show them what our medicines can do, prescribed according to our laws?

Let me repeat. A girl suffering for thirteen years from a disfiguring skin disease, told by a leading specialist that nothing more could be done for her, 'she would have to put up with it', improved rapidly from the moment she received treatment on Hahnemannian lines. *Graphites* which is black lead as used for drawing pencils, produces tetters and eczema, if taken in large doses and cures it if a similar eruption is found in sick people, rapidly and painlessly. My patient was kept under observation for five years and only showed slight recurrences after months of being free from any blemish and these were always rapidly controlled by a few doses of her remedy. And again, in impetigo, which requires months of treatment and months of exclusion from school sometimes as it is so contagious; this can be controlled and cured with very little bother with *Tartar Emetic* in little over a week.

Chicken-pox, which has a similar encrusted pustular eruption, disappears in a few days without leaving scars or pitting due to the irritation of the rash and the scratching and picking of the sufferer. Chicken-pox is said to be a mild disease, not needing medical attention. How disastrous the consequences can be, if chicken-pox is neglected! A little girl died last week of the after-effects of chicken-pox; she had never been well since her attack in February and had been continually under medical treatment after the pocks had disappeared, as she felt and looked so ill. She was never 'diagnosed', only iron tonics and malt were given, and when she landed in hospital she died after two days. When a post-mortem examination was made she was found to be suffering from tubercular meningitis. She was undoubtedly a victim of the war and the evacuation scheme; for while she was under homoeopathic treatment until last summer, although she was thin and had been delicate and slow at first in putting on weight, was getting on satisfactorily. She had gained on *Tuberculinum* and in June, 1939, she was given *Drosera* and had done very nicely by the end of July. Then her parents sent her to Devon in September and she was seen again early in December, when she had done remarkably well. She went back to the West of England, developed chicken-pox which was neglected and then the latent tuberculosis showed itself and killed her. It shows, alas, that *Drosera*, as already stated by Hahnemann, is closely related to tuber-culosis, the disease was held at bay while the child was under its influence; when removed from homoeopathic treatment she died from the disease, though until chicken-pox developed, she appeared to be well, and had been gaining weight rapidly.

Quel dommage! I recall a similar case of severe chicken-pox, the child looked collapsed and alarmingly ill; he had had high fever round 103°-104° for ten days under allopathic treatment, and looked ready for the undertaker when I saw him. He was given *Silica* and a week later *Drosera*, and he flourished after that.

'Skins' do well on homoeopathic treatment, though on occasions the process of curing may severely tax the patience of the sufferer and demand the greatest skill and knowledge on the part of the doctor.

CHAPTER EIGHTEEN

SOME COMPLICATIONS OF
INFECTIOUS DISEASES

Infectious diseases are accountable for a large amount of illness among children and even adults; unfortunately most cases of infectious diseases are segregated in fever hospitals by the local municipal authorities and the homoeopathic general practitioner gets very little opportunity of trying out what his little pills can do — *unless* he ignores the law and by not notifying the respective infectious disease, keeps the case at home. If he has the necessary knowledge and the courage of his convictions he will cure the child in a minimum of time and without any of the serious sequelae which follow so frequently after orthodox treatment. I have proved the truth of this statement again and again in the past; now I do not often see the cases in the acute stages, I only see the after effects. How often does one hear this: 'the child has never been well since an attack of Scarlet Fever or Diphtheria.'

Post-measles or post-scarlatinal debility, heart trouble or debility is common, and the usual treatment is: Change of air, convalescence which has to be paid for by local charitable societies; or if the debility is not so serious, a course of iron pills or iron mixture, or some similar 'tonic' is advised.

I saw such a child some time ago, on January 28th, 1937, she was then twelve years old, a thin, pallid child, brought to me for a cough — a deep dry cough which came mainly from the stomach. She was always tired, always lazy, did not want to do anything, did not want to go out, did not want to play even. Had heart trouble after scarlet fever in May, 1935, had not been the same since. On examination the heart was found to be somewhat dilated, the second sound in the mitral area was accentuated, she was white and pallid though her lips were red.

Her weight was 5 st. 8 lb. 12 oz. She was given *Sulph.* 30

on her tiredness and her general appearance, and told to rest in bed.

On February 11th, 1937, the report was: Still very tired, changeable, complains of tiredness on walking fast, and the mother again emphasized the fact that she had never been well since the attack of scarlet fever. *Thuja* 30.

February 18th. Better this week, not so tired, worries about going back to school. Weight 5 st. 10 lb. 12 oz. – a gain of 2 lb.

March 4th. Less tired, eating better. To be excluded from school for another few weeks. *Thuja* 30.

March 18th. Better, eating better; to continue resting – does not complain now about walking too fast.

Weight 5 st. 13 lb. 8 oz. – a gain of nearly 5 lb. in six weeks. This was due to rest and the correctly indicated medicine which improved the metabolism. There was no change made in her diet. Poor people cannot afford extra milk and eggs for the children.

April 8th, 1937. Better, more like her old self, no shortness of breath now, much better colour, heart not dilated, sounds normal. To return to school. Weight 6 st. *Thuja* 30.

I did not see her again until thirteen months later, on May 12th, 1938, when she was brought for a cough after swimming. Her first period came on in December, 1937, and lasted one week, no periods since. *Puls.* 30 t.d.s.

May 19th, 1938. Better. Weight 6 st. 10 lb., gained 10 lb. since 8.4.37, and over 15 lb. since January 28th, 1937, that is in not quite sixteen months. *Sulph.* 30.

July 19th, 1938. The mother stopped me in the street to tell me how well the child was, and that her periods were now regular.

September 15th, 1938. Brought for a sore throat. Ulcers on both tonsils, better for hot drinks; sore throat started on right side and went over to the left side, pain worse on empty swallowing – heart nothing abnormal, has been in bed for two days. *Lycopodium* 30.

September 22nd, 1938. Cold gone, throat cleared up in

twenty-four hours after the medicine, feels well in herself.

Weight 7 st. 4 lb. 8 oz., a gain of 1 st. 9¾ lb. from the end of January, 1937, to the end of September, 1938, that is in one year and eight months. An excellent record, if you take into consideration that the child lived in a working-class neighbourhood of London, that she did not have any change of air during the whole of this time, and that her diet was the ordinary diet of a working-class home. And for two years previously she had been ailing, never felt well, had no appetite, had not got on in school.

The only addition that was made was some homoeopathic medication, a few doses of *Sulphur* and *Thuja*.

Was this just accidental? The mother knew better, she gave the praise to the treatment received, 'the wonderful pills she had been having', as she called it. A much cheaper way than sending a child away for weeks to a convalescent home. What a lot of public money could be saved, if only doctors would get to know about homoeopathy and would trouble to apply it and not scorn it.

Now, another case of complication after measles in December, 1935, followed by a discharging ear, for a whole month. First seen on January 23rd, 1936. Perforated right ear, very spoilt, faddy child, does not like fat, cries all the time, wants a lot of fuss made of him. *Pulsatilla* 30 given on the general indications. The ear cleared up within two weeks after the *Pulsatilla*.

On June 24th, 1937, he was seen again for 'rough spots underneath the skin of his face'. Right ear was dry and there was scarring over the perforation of the drum, a pigmented 'spider naevus' underneath right eye. *Thuja* 30. No local treatment for spots which disappeared in a few days.

July 11th, 1938. Came this time for severe haemorrhage after dental extraction and ulcerative stomatitis. The mouth was extremely offensive and inflamed, the sockets of the teeth were inflamed, tongue coated, the breath foul. Temperature 99.8° — the right drum was sound, and the naevus noticed thirteen months ago on his face had disappeared — without local treatment.

He was given *Mercurius* 30 night and morning for three days.

Seen two days later, the mouth was sweet and clean, the ulcers had disappeared and there was no inflammation of the gums. No mouth-wash was given, no local treatment was ordered. Homoeopathy works rapidly, provided you get the correct remedies.

I was interested also in this last case to make the observation that the naevus on the child's right cheek disappeared after the *Thuja*.

A naevus is said to be due to delayed vaccinal poisoning, which may appear in children of over-vaccinated parents; whether this is so or not, the fact remains that *Thuja* in this instance removed the naevus. And *Thuja* is the generally recognized antidote for vaccinosis. I do not know how long *Thuja* took to cure the naevus. I did not see the child often enough to watch it carefully, but in a little over a year it had completely gone. And the foul discharge from the ear which came on after measles dried up in a week or two after *Pulsatilla*, the remedy indicated by the characteristics of the little boy. I have known these cases of purulent ear discharge after measles go on for years and years, and they could be stopped, if taken in hand early, and much unnecessary suffering could be saved.

Diphtheria is another disease which leads to subsequent ill-health; whether this is due to the treatment received in the hospitals or due to the toxins remaining in the blood-stream, is a moot question, and more than probably this disease, if treated homoeopathically, would not lead to heart disease and paralysis. Nervous disabilities are often left behind after diphtheria. I remember a young woman who had a short, sharp attack of diphtheria for which she received the orthodox treatment in the fever hospital — that is diphtheria antitoxin injections. It cured the diphtheria, but she never felt well afterwards. She used to be in the best of health before, except she was inclined to be afflicted with a slight inferiority complex. Her brothers and sisters were so much cleverer than she was; she was the dunce of the family, she considered. This feeling of inferiority grew and grew after her discharge from the fever hospital. She developed almost immediately severe brachial neuritis of the left arm. She lost weight, became white and pale, and full of nervous fears and obsessions. She was terrified of doctors, she got into frightful states of agitation, before going to hospital or going to her panel doctor, her hands used to shake and tremble. She could not open her mouth to speak, her tongue clove to her palate with fright, she perspired all over from sheer funk and scare. No doctor could get anything out of her. She was sent into a nerve hospital, but she could not stand the sight of the other patients, they only made her worse. Her agitation became worse, her eyes were staring out of her head, and she looked wild, her husband and parents could do nothing with her. Strangers agitated her, she even threatened to commit suicide, as she was a disgrace to her family and a drag on her husband.

When I saw her she was a pitiful nervous wreck. She was now thirty-three years of age and had not been well for eleven years, since she had this attack of diphtheria; she was very definite about this history of ill-health since diphtheria. Always septic fingers and septic throats for the last eleven years — nature's attempt of getting rid of the antitoxin poison which had been injected into the blood-stream. Pains in the neck and chest, feeling of tightness round the chest, severe rheumatic pains in the legs and feet, and then this agonizing neuritis in the left arm, the great depression, always weeping, feels hopeless, does not like gloomy weather, timid, shy and emotional, and feels better for sympathy.

It took me a very long time to get anything out of her; she was in such a state of fear and agitation. I prescribed *Pulsatilla* 6, three times daily, and asked her to come back in a month.

Seen again on November 29th, 1937, she still feels very depressed, feels she is never going to get better, still afraid to speak, has had some days during the last month when she felt she was going to improve.

Has been vaccinated twice, did not take the second time.

She was not quite so terror-stricken this time, got her words out with rather an effort and long pauses in between. Told me she had been attending three different hospitals, gone from place to place, and nobody seemed to understand her. Everything was put down to nerves and she was told to pull herself together. She pathetically remarked, she had tried so hard and could not manage it somehow. She wished somebody would tell her how.

As an antidote against repeated vaccinations she was given *Thuja* 30, to be followed by *Phosphorus* 30 for her various fears. She was afraid of being attacked by consumption, afraid of storms, and liked to be made a fuss of.

Seen January 6th, 1938. Complains of tightness of chest, does not feel nearly so depressed or weepy, has more rheumatism, intercostal muscles thickened, also thickening of left sterno-mastoid. *Thuja* 30.

February 19th, 1938. Much better. Weight is 8 st. 4 lb., a gain of 6 lb. since her first visit on October 30th, 1937. She had been put on a fattening diet, more milk, one egg daily, more butter, more sugar such as barley sugar, and brown demerara sugar. And she has responded well.

Indigestion much better, depression much improved, feeling of weight and of an iron band round the chest gone. Sleeping well, has no troublesome dreams now. Still shakes and trembles on coming here, and complains of lack of confidence. Feels the cold very much. To continue *Thuja*.

May 10th, 1938. More like herself in every way. Not so many fears, not afraid of dark, of being alone, or of thunderstorms now, not afraid of 'developing consumption' any more. Used to have a sick feeling in the streets, fear of falling down, all this has gone. *Thuja* 1m.

July 11th, 1938. Weight 8 st. 5 lb. No fears, much steadier here, talks freely now, eyes steady, do not look so wild or staring. Pain in the left arm and neck much about the same. I told her that these pains would be the last to go; the greatest improvement being in her mind, the physical symptoms would go, too, in due course.

September 7th, 1938. Weight 8 st. 6 lb., looks well and

feels well. Has had a holiday at the seaside, and everybody remarked how different her behaviour was. She could mix freely with strangers now, could enjoy a joke, she walked for miles without getting tired. She is just her normal self — happy, contented and serene. Her husband is so delighted that she has been saved from the asylum. They were all afraid she was going insane, as she was so peculiar.

Has had some indigestion while she was on holiday. She cannot digest fat or cream. Ordered *Puls.* 1*m*.

This lady suffered from fears following after anti-diphtheria serum injections, and poisoning from repeated vaccinations.

Once these animal toxins were antidoted, her metabolism improved, she was able to throw off her nervous fears and tremors, and become normal once more.

Where would she have ended otherwise? For she contemplated suicide. Homoeopathy saved her! And yet the majority of the medical profession persist in saying that diphtheria antitoxin does not harm, that vaccination with calf lymph is necessary and leaves no trace in the human body.

Again and again one finds that mysterious illnesses following vaccination, immunization and antitoxine treatments are cleared up when the right homoeopathic remedies are used.

CHAPTER NINETEEN

IMMUNIZATION

For years I have been considering the subject of immunization against Diphtheria; for the prevention of any disease — especially of diphtheria — is to the healer a grand and worthwhile project. This particular infectious disease is the most treacherous of all. Like a thunderbolt out of the blue it strikes down its victim; an only child seems to be its special prey. Its death rate was very high in the past; for the last thirty years or so it has dropped considerably all over the country and I believe all over the globe.

I was early introduced to the terror of diphtheria. This was a playmate of mine who had joined in our games at her birthday party the day before; death plucked her out of our midst, and she was dead twenty-four hours later. And she was the only one infected. The why and wherefore remained a mystery.

Diphtheria is therefore a disease to be dreaded, and one is only too willing to advocate anything and to try out anything which promises to be a cure, and what is better still, promises to prevent this disease.

Antitoxin was introduced as a curative measure and was said to give a high percentage of cures, if given early in large enough doses. And now within the last fifteen years this new idea of immunization has come over from the States and Canada, which claims that inoculation against diphtheria has practically wiped out this disease in the State of New York ever since general inoculation was introduced.

On studying the statistics of the death rate in New York, one sees that the fall in the diphtheria death rate was much greater in the years preceding the introduction of immunization than it was afterwards.

This natural decline in the death rate was due to other

factors, namely, this disease, like all the infectious diseases, goes through different cycles of high and low virulence, and this low virulence type of diphtheria set in before immunization was carried out, and was therefore not due to it; and the lowered death rate was just a lucky coincidence.

Now diphtheria immunization has been strictly enforced by the health authorities in Germany with the result that this disease has increased from 46,905 cases in 1928, to 149,490 in 1938 — the last year for which figures are available; an increase of over 100,000 per year, in spite of, or is it because of the immunization? This means number of people attacked, not the number who died. No figures for this are available, as far as I know.

In Sweden, on the other hand, not a single death from diphtheria has been recorded for the last three years though immunization has not been resorted to except in isolated cases.

Does this speak well for the contention that immunization prevents diphtheria?

In Great Britain the number of fully immunized children who have developed diphtheria in spite of it, has gone up considerably. Published figures in Eire and some large towns in England, show that over 3,000 cases of failure to protect against diphtheria have been recorded and out of this number 50 have died.

And how does the saga go? Immunization protects against diphtheria; and if the child should be so unlucky as to be attacked by it, it will only be of a mild type! Can somebody tell me, if it is only a mild type of disease, why did 50 cases die of it?

Now it has been proved many times that immunized children not only become more sensitive to diphtheria for the first six months after inoculation, but that a good many of them become carriers of the disease after immunization. They are therefore a danger to others.

It was mentioned in one of the broadcasts lately that inoculation 'does not upset a child in the least'. Now medical officers and manufacturing chemists speak freely and openly about the greater or lesser liability of the different products used for inoculation in causing 'reactions' which include pain, swelling, nausea, malaise, rise of temperature and a general feeling of illness for several days.

This is the immediate reaction which is something that is not denied by either doctors or laboratory workers, or chemical manufacturers. The more remote effects, such as loss of weight, general debility, weakness, and other complications are frequently ignored.

Has the harmlessness of the procedure really been proved? What about the tuberculosis which developed in nearly all the children who were immunized at a public institution in Lübeck, North Germany, a few years ago?

What about the case of the child who developed tuberculosis after inoculation in Eire and died of it not so long ago? The fact that tuberculosis had developed was never denied before the magistrate; but nobody would bear the onus. The manufacturers declared that no accident could have happened in their laboratories; they were fool-proof. The inoculating doctor declared that he had used the right inoculating tube in a manner advised by the firm of well-known makers, and in the end, it was found to be an act of God, and the matter was left in abeyance.

As I have said before, I was willing to co-operate in any treatment which set out to prevent diphtheria. With an open mind I stood by for several years, being in the fortunate position of a Medical Officer at two clinics which boasted an immunization centre, I was able to watch and see the children before and after inoculation. Right early on, some years ago, there was a child who immediately after an attack of diphtheria was immunized at the Fever Hospital. She had been a healthy child before; normal in weight and development; but after this all growth ceased; she remained a puny, delicate, and ailing child; it was so pronounced that she was a byword in the whole neighbourhood and for years not a single parent in that street would consent to have a child of theirs inoculated.

A year or so later I saw another child who had been

inoculated; again the same thing happened, growth and progress ceased, no gain in weight; she was very anaemic and bloodless, almost as white as a lily. She was given Parrish's food at hospital, she was sent away on convalescence for eight weeks; then a little while later she went to the sea-side for four weeks or so. This went on for years and the last time I heard about her, just before the war started, she had been away at a school camp for over six months; but I could not find any improvement. She cost the ratepayers and charitable institutions a pretty penny.

There were altogether some half-a-dozen similar cases in this immediate neighbourhood, who became weakly and ailing and 'bad doers' after immunization; and practically every child I saw after it had been inoculated seemed to come to a standstill, inoculation seemed to check general progress for a considerable period. No wonder I was not very enthusiastic after such experiences.

Three adults, all of them nurses, offered themselves for inoculation in order to prove to the mothers that the operation was painless and harmless. All three had to go off duty; all three had swollen and painful arms and were ill in bed for several days with high temperatures ranging between 101° and 103°. Two of them refused the second inoculation, as it made them too ill; the third bravely carried on, and once more she was on a bed of sickness for nearly a week.

Then the most tragic of all the cases: a pretty little girl of ten, who had never had a day's illness previously, developed general blood poisoning after immunization and died three months later.

No, it is not correct to say that this practice is harmless in all cases; far from it.

Does immunization protect against diphtheria? One doctor's son I knew, was inoculated and had to be sent to the Fever Hospital within a month suffering from diphtheria.

And, unfortunately, apparently for six months after inoculation you must not go near anybody who is a carrier or who has got diphtheria, as you get more sensitive to the infection during that period.

Another child who had been fully immunized and given a

certificate to that effect, seven months afterwards, after the so-called negative phase had passed, developed diphtheria and died within twelve hours of the fulminating type of this disease. And yet you are told, even if attacked, you will only have a mild type of diphtheria!

On comparing notes with the M.O. of one of the Immunization Clinics, I was told that these accidents were due to the particular variety of immunizing agent used; in his clinic, on the other hand, they used another variety, and no accidents like that ever happened; he had no failures.

He spoke too soon, a couple of months later one of his successes developed diphtheria and at least two other children developed marasmus and remained weakly and delicate.

And, do you know, he did not come near me for several months afterwards!

The proposition that diphtheria can be prevented by inoculation sounds attractive in theory, but does not work out so nicely in practice; neither is there any agreement between immunizing doctors as regards the kind of immunizing agent to be used, the number of doses required, and the length of time immunity will hold good and how often therefore re-inoculation is necessary.

Everything is still in a state of flux and in the experimental stage, and therefore not only inexact but unscientific. But it involves more than a question of the amount to be inoculated in one or two or three doses. After all, what is inoculation but the injection of products of diphtheria into the blood stream and the tissues, and therefore it should not be permitted.

Do you realize that the serum is not even human serum, but is made by being passed through an animal body, it may be a horse, a guinea-pig, or a rabbit; and that animal serums do not really harmonize with human serum.

Now life is really a question of electrical radiations between and within the cells. When radiation ceases, life is at an end; the radiations in a human being whose normal span of life is three score and ten, are at a totally different wavelength from those of a guinea-pig, for example, whose life is a matter of months, not years; or even those of a horse which lives perhaps 20-24 years. Consider what happens when you place an electric bulb for 120 volts in a circuit which works at 240 volts; there is a flash, a fuse and the lamp will be broken. The same happens in the human body when animal serum is mixed with it. You get a shock, a lowering of blood-pressure, faintness, even collapse and in some cases sudden death. It may not happen the first time; but in cases of repeated inoculations, as is the fashion now of injecting serums for all sorts of diseases, you run the risk of causing serious shocks.

Yes, on due consideration I have come to the conclusion that immunization with animal diphtheria serum or any other serum is bad; the dosage is too large, and the results are too uncertain, also, from a humanitarian point of view it is wrong.

What do homoeopaths want immunizing substances for? We have got much better agents which have been used clinically and proved many years before immunization was even thought of. We call them nosodes; they are not made by being passed through animal bodies, so no needless suffering is caused to our younger brothers of the animal world, which I am sure is not right from the humanitarian and spiritual standpoint.

No, the nosodes are made in the same way as all our other remedies: diluted on the centesimal scale; well shaken up and succussed and thus potentised, made more active, until a high stage of power is reached, and the latent energies in each drug are released. Our medium and high potencies have a dynamic action, not a chemical or a physiological one. It is no good at all to give these nosodes in the low potencies, they would just reproduce the disease; but given in unit doses in a high potency at long intervals, they do what they set out to do, they make a person immune to that particular disease. Do you remember in the January, 1939, number of 'HEAL THYSELF' Dr. Schmidt mentioning the experiments done by Dr. Cherrian of Paris, with *Diphtherinum* on animals and on humans. He inoculated animals, pigs, hens and other beasties against diphtheria by giving them the nosode of *Diphtherinum* in the 4*m* and the 8*m* potency and obtained protection after only one dose of this high potency for five to six years.

I have given *Diphtherinum* in the 200th potency in several cases and so far I have not heard of any case of diphtheria developing; no failure so far, and no severe reactions followed, no wasting, no debility, such as I have described following on the overdosing by the strong allopathic diphtheria serum. No, remember the risks of accidents which are one of the snags of every form of crude immunization, as urged by the orthodox school.

Compulsory immunization is a dangerous practice and the present campaign should be strongly opposed by all followers of the homoeopathic teachings.

Diphtheria is largely a matter of public sanitation. Improved drainage and clean water supply will reduce the incidence of diphtheria. Diphtheria is a dirt disease, a disease due to neglect of the laws of hygiene, which were propounded by Moses in the Old Testament. You will never get rid of diphtheria by pumping products of the disease into the system; you will only get further and worse disease. Follow the natural laws of health, keep yourself well by simple living, by drinking clean water, by eating clean, unadulterated food and thus building up a strong, healthy soil in your body which will then be able to resist all disease germs. It is the old, old story which can never be emphasized enough. Live on a well selected diet, clean milk, home made cream cheese, in short on a lacto-vegetarian diet containing a mixture of properly cooked or steamed and raw vegetables, and wholemeal bread which has not been robbed of its wheat germ and its bran, adding small quantities of meat, poultry and fish, should you feel so disposed. Never mind all this scientific jargon of vitamins; this diet will have all the vitamins you require. And thus fortified, you will not need to fear diphtheria or any other bogey disease with which the orthodox fraternity may like to frighten you.

CHAPTER TWENTY

ON THE PREVENTION OF DISEASE

Influenza is a word that is often taken in vain and used by some people to describe any and every feverish chill which may attack them. But should you be seized by this enemy you will indeed know it. It leaves in its wake a feeling of utter weariness, exhaustion, prostration and limpness, even though there may only have been a day or two of rise of temperature. It is a general nerve poison and it has, like most illnesses, a special rhythm of its own. It breaks out every twenty weeks or so and should this outbreak coincide with the season of inclement weather, you will get a lesser or larger epidemic, according to the number attacked. That is why you hear more of influenza in the winter months. Every few years the influenza virus seems to become specially active, indeed it has been shown that every thirty years a general pandemic sweeps the world. That was so in the years 1888-90 and again in 1918-19; during those years thousands and tens of thousands died of this disease, both in the temperate climes and in the tropics.

There has not been any severe or prolonged outbreak of influenza in 1948-49, thus missing the 30 year cycle of return of this pandemic. My theory is, and it's as good as anybody else's, (1) that the consumption of meat and other nitrogenous products has been lowered owing to circumstances beyond our control (2) the increased consumption of salads, raw and cooked vegetables and potatoes, and a higher extraction rate of bread which contains more roughage.

The bacteriologists are very troubled, they have been hunting this evasive bug for years and never found it yet. Now and again you read in the papers that influenza is conquered, that a distinguished laboratory worker has found the cause at last; and now a cure is certain! But still influenza goes on merrily and leads all the bacteriologists a dance, like the will-o'-the-wisp. They have made up different varieties of vaccines and serums, without avail, but the death-rate remains high. All the immunity which can be promised is, that if you are inoculated in the autumn, there will be, perhaps, a certain safety period for 6-8 weeks. I think that this is the latest verdict. Of course, the well-vaunted Sulphonamides, the latest cure-all, are said to help you over an attack rapidly, but, I am afraid, it has already ceased to live up to its reputation. It seems to bring the temperature down with a vengeance, only to be followed in a certain number of cases by various complications and sudden inexplicable deaths.

I heard of a young woman who had caught a very powerful germ, as she put it, which had given her pink eye, bronchitis, urticaria, a high temperature for over a fortnight, and she was still as bad as ever. It does not say much for modern treatment, does it? Germs are scavengers and would never do any damage unless they found a suitable soil to thrive in.

Prevention really boils itself down again to obeying the simple rules of health; living on simple food, as much as possible, largely on fruits of the field and meadows and gardens, that is, on fresh vegetables, properly cooked and prepared; on raw fruits, on wholemeal bread which should contain the wheat germ and the bran — on milk, pure, clean unadulterated milk — on such milk products as cheese and butter — and meat and fish only in the smallest quantities for those that cannot do without its stimulating properties. Fresh fruits, lemons, limes, oranges, grapefruit and pineapples are store-houses of sunshine, so deficient for many months in these misty sea-girt islands. They contain the essential vitamin C which prevents scurvy, and besides this they also contain, which I think even more important, the necessary mineral salts in an organic form, salts which make and keep the blood stream alkaline and are necessary to keep the metabolism going and the composition of the blood stream pure. Influenza is a disease during which a wastage of the mineral salts takes place and in order to recover from an attack rapidly, you should live on an eliminating diet, a diet which cleans and purifies and throws the minimum amount of work on the digestive organs. The juice of oranges and lemons does all that, pleasantly and easily, much better than such so-called strengthening foods as meat-juices, and clogging drinks as milk.

I have found during many years of experience that an orange diet for several days in influenza, or indeed most feverish illnesses, whether infectious or not, will rapidly bring the temperature down and the patient after a few days on fruit juices will experience a feeling of internal cleanness and arise refreshed without any feeling of prostration, so that convalescence is a matter of days instead of weeks or even months. Unfortunately I have already noticed that where there is an absence of citrus fruit, influenza seems to drag on, even though the temperature comes down rapidly with the correctly prescribed remedy, there are more unpleasant complications than I ever experienced before; and many dozens of cases have been through my hands in the 1918 epidemic and since.

Have you noticed that all the fruit and vegetables which contain vitamin C and are therefore stores of sunshine, are either bright yellow or orange? If there is anything in colour therapy, this is another proof of its value. Swedes and carrots contain vitamin C as well. Swedes are roots which grow above ground and get plenty of sun; but it is difficult to extract the juice without a special machine. We tried it in the last war and what a nuisance it was! Tomatoes, too, are a lovely orange colour and contain a quantity of vitamin C. There is another vegetable, very little known in this country; the Hungarian sweet pepper or paprika, which is a mild cayenne, and is again of a lovely orange-red colour; this grows and ripens in the sun-drenched steppes of Hungary, having been kissed by the rays of the sun, it is full of vitamin C. It is sold in this country as a fine reddish powder and if and when obtainable, should be used to replace the missing oranges and lemons, making a very tasty addition to soups, stews, sauces for vegetables, or it may be simply added to hot milk. It is the sauce piquante of the high-class chef.

They offer you all kinds of artificial substitutes for vitamin C now, but I for one am chary of using or ordering the artificial chemicals, concentrated products of the art of the laboratory-worker, which some scientific or pseudo-scientific advisers of the Ministry of Health have strongly recommended should be added to margarine, bread and other vital necessities of life. Only relatively minute quantities of vitamins are necessary; and the quantities of vitamin consumed by some people in bread, etc., might be very large, their action on the human system is unknown, and they could do untold damage, and might well produce some new puzzling forms of disease. Diseases do change with each decade; even in the lower kingdoms the same is taking place. Until the last twenty years or so, in gardening and agriculture natural manures were generally used, these have been more and more replaced by artificial fertilizers, owing to the shortage of horse, cow and pig manure. These artificial, concentrated, inorganic mineral salts were being added to the soil, and at first appeared to act wonderfully well, growth was more luxuriant, fruit and vegetables increased in size, colours were more vivid, but — and this is a big but — gradually more and more bacterial diseases were showing themselves; more parasites became evident, there was the antirrhinum disease, there arose the strawberry blight which nearly decimated whole fields in the South of England; the phylloxera disease of vine, etc., and the number of chemical sprays are now increasing year by year to combat this invasion of parasites, big and small, and to antidote the bacterial infections. And surely, chemical sprays cannot be good, if the plants are grown for human consumption?

Again the quality of fruit and vegetables has deteriorated at the same time; they are larger but tasteless and lacking in flavour. I had noticed for years that vegetables and also fruit tasted insipid and had lost everything which made them interesting. I put it down for a time to my advancing years and that I was approaching the time of life when all enjoyment in food was lost; that the flavour of youth had gone. But latterly I have tasted vegetables which have been grown without artificial manures, on soil which had been properly enriched by suitably prepared compost heaps according to the Rudolf Steiner and similar methods, and all at once I rediscovered the old flavour of vegetables of my younger days. So the fault lay in the coarse, overgrown, wrongly-manured vegetables, not in me. These tasteless vegetables are the reason why British people add such huge amounts of condiments to their food in order to make it palatable; too much salt, pepper and mustard are bad for the liver, kidneys and digestive organs, if people would only realize it.

Now vegetables grown on healthy soil, made healthy by adding compost from vegetable waste, no longer develop parasitical diseases, no longer require spraying as has been proved by trial over a number of years by many gardeners and farmers.

The compost is made by placing all vegetable refuse such as weeds, nettles, bracken, cut grass, spent annuals and vegetable leaves into a heap or heaps. All is of use except dry sticks and autumn leaves which should be formed into a separate heap. There are various methods recommended in building these up according to different authorities. The one I like best is known as Q.R., which was developed by the late Miss May Bruce of Cirencester, Glos. She used a special activator made up of Chamomile, Dandelion, Nettle, Yarrow, Valerian, powdered oak bark and pure run Honey. I found this activator worked well in reducing a compost heap into a friable, sweet-smelling soil. Artificial fertilizers, whatever their chemical stimulants, act like allopathic medicines, producing over-stimulation, the plants being weak and an easy prey to disease caused by parasites and different viruses. This very effective compost maker can be obtained in powder form with full instructions for preparation from very many seed merchants and horticulturists at a moderate price. As it is entirely herbal in origin, it is of particular value to those who appreciate natural methods.

It is essential the health of the nation should be preserved;

174 *More Magic of the Minimum Dose*

we have got to live simply, and live on the products of the earth, and therefore proper methods should be made known and broadcast so that the keen gardeners can produce the healthiest, best-tasting vegetables possible. Fertile soil is of the greatest importance, soil is not just a chemical factory, and growth does not depend alone on automatic chemical changes. Growth is made possible by living forces and radiations inherent at different wavelengths in each member of the four kingdoms, mineral (stones), vegetable, animal and human.

I strongly believe, as I have said before that you should not introduce a foreign rhythm of life from the animal world into the human world, or from the animal world into the plant world, or from the mineral into the plant kingdom. It produces a disturbance of vibrations and radiations and produces disease; hence plant diseases follow the use of artificial mineral manures. The plants grown on a living fertile soil made active by the interplay of living forces from the vegetable kingdom thrive under the health-giving rays of the sun and the drenching rain, and store up power and energy and in due season are ready to be consumed by and taken up into the living human factory, there to revitalize and renew it. Vegetables and corn are best for growth, better than meat and fish. Remember the story in the Old Testament when Daniel as a young lad refused to eat the king's meat and drink the king's wine, and begged to be allowed to live on vegetables, pulses and the like, and to drink only water. The royal steward who was responsible to King Nebuchadnezzar for the well-being of this school of young Jewish nobles was doubtful about it, but consented to try this vegetable diet for ten days and after that time it was found that the children fed on vegetables were fatter and their countenances appeared fairer than the children fed on a meat and wine diet. Thus the steward became convinced and continued feeding them on vegetables and pulses to their immeasurable benefit.

I wonder whether any still remember the chatty books of Mrs. Earle's on Gardening and allied subjects, vegetables, cooking, health, history; everything was discussed. She was asked by a friend whether she was not afraid of living out in the country so far away from the amenities of towns; what would she do if she ever became ill, especially as the doctor lived miles away from her house. 'Why,' Mrs. Earle replied, 'What should I want a doctor for; I am always well, I live on vegetables and fruit only, and never get influenza or any other acute disease.' Mrs. Earle died only a few short years ago, well past the scriptural age of seventy years — well over eighty, if my memory serves me right.

Yes, if people would only remember that germs do not matter, diseases are to a large extent our own fault, and what is of the greatest importance is to keep the soil in good heart, to refertilize the soil of Britain in the right way and then valuable human lives will be saved. I heard a doctor holding forth on bacteria and germs today, drawing lurid tales about the multitude of them and frightening or trying to frighten his listeners with the damage these could do. I wish doctors for a change would leave bacteria alone and make people health conscious, by insisting that health can be restored and kept by living on pure, unspoilt, fresh and unadulterated food, such as vegetables and fruit, plus milk, fresh cream, cheese, eggs and wholesome unfortified, unprocessed wholemeal bread, not forgetting pure cane-sugar and English honey.

But our food must not be interfered with, nothing must be subtracted, nothing added; the milk must be fresh from healthy cows and unpasteurised, for if the cows are kept clean and milked by milkers who know the value of clean udders and clean hands, there will be little bacterial growth and there will be no need to kill bacteria which are not there, by pasteurizing the milk. Make the cows free from tubercular infection, by feeding them on compost grown grass, without artificial manures, and if necessary giving those already infected a course of our *Tuberculinum* over a few months. Our cattle would be able to stand up better to all kinds of diseases, such as mastitis, contagious abortion, foot and mouth disease, etc., which can and should be cured by homoeopathy. But our masters start at the wrong end of the stick, they medicate our food, which is grown on unnatural soil, richly dosed with all kinds of inorganic mineral salts — medicines again — and the results are: a C3 nation lacking in energy, lacking in initiative, willing, even anxious, to give up all its liberties, handed down by their sturdy ancestors, the yeomen of England. I repeat it — a C3 nation, under the heel of a vast bureaucratic National Health Service — the irony of it!

CHAPTER TWENTY-ONE

DIPHTHERIA AND ITS NOSODE

In the temperate part of the hemisphere winter has been and always will be a period of danger for such diseases as influenza, catarrhal troubles, feverish chills and infectious diseases. The more thoughtful of the population have been considering how to avert and prevent many of these ailments, which are made worse by over-crowding, huddling together in badly ventilated and concreted shelters. Fortunately the croakers who prophesied much illness during the first eighteen months of the war have been proved wrong; maybe this is due largely to people being too busy and getting on with their jobs, and the other important cause of comparatively little illness is due to simpler feeding, the eating of less sugar and sweets, and the compulsory consumption of less meat per person, for sugar, specially beet sugar, increases catarrhal troubles.

I saw in a daily paper in the late autumn an article on the prevention of winter ills written by an orthodox doctor, who was of the opinion that shortly it would be possible to stamp out practically all of the infectious diseases which sweep through towns and country places year after year. And how does he suggest this should be done? He says that the individuals can help themselves to health and thus benefit the whole community by reinforcing their own natural resistance to the majority of ailments by vaccination and inoculation.

He argues that most people who have had a particular infectious disease, are immune to that disease or in common parlance, are not likely to suffer from that fever again, as one attack causes nature to produce in our bloodstreams certain anti-bodies, which act as powerful defensive agents against a renewed assault by that particular germ.

He also states that in some of the infectious diseases it is not necessary to wait for the attacking enemy to develop the necessary resistance, and that this resistance can be artificially produced by injecting or inoculating a serum or vaccine.

Then he draws up a chart for certain of the infectious diseases, which I shall copy and then make a few explanatory remarks so as to refute some of his statements.

This doctor is honest in some of his statements; most authorities claim 100 per cent protection against diphtheria and suppress the fact that at least 25 per cent of the inoculated children are attacked by diphtheria. He, however, makes a bad mistake in saying that there is no reaction or only a very slight reaction in a child after inoculation. I have seen the arm swell up from the shoulder right down to the wrist; I have seen high temperatures lasting for 4-5 days; and I have seen remote effects lasting for years, until they were antidoted by either *Thuja* or *Pulsatilla*. Such effects as severe anaemia, weakness, tiredness, loss of weight, the child remaining undersized and delicate, not able to stand up to the overcrowding of city life, with some improvement in the country, and immediately slipping back and losing six or seven lb. on return to town life. As soon as one or two doses of *Thuja* were given in the 30th or 200th potency, everything improved, sometimes it had to be followed up and the results were better with *Pulsatilla* 6 or 12, 2-3 times daily. Even with adults one noted a lack of the joy of life, a disinclination to work, a dragging round slowly and laboriously; with a return to the normal zest of life when *Pulsatilla* or *Thuja* was given.

Disease	Chances of gaining protection		Method used	Time of treatment and approximate number of of injections	
Diphtheria	75%	There is usually a complete immunity	Injection	2 doses 4 weeks apart	(See Remarks)

As for saying that the protection would last probably for life, nobody can say that for certain, as immunization is too recent an experiment; or did the doctor mean for life, if life was shortened by an attack of diphtheria?

Compulsory diphtheria inoculation was introduced into Germany in the 1920s and yet Germany has the second highest incidence rate of diphtheria in Europe. There were 1,500 deaths from diphtheria in Germany in 1926 and in 1937 the deaths from diphtheria had risen to 5,400. In 1923 France had 11,033 cases of diphtheria; in 1930 after a general propaganda campaign for immunization there were 23,704 cases notified; while Sweden without immunization had 113 cases of diphtheria without any deaths in 1938.

Is diphtheria really so prevalent and the danger to the general population as great as it is made out to be? A headmaster who managed a boarding school for 300 boys for 27 years states that there never was a single case of diphtheria among all his boys during the whole of that period. I should say, this was due to the excellent sanitation and water supply of that school and to proper feeding and the healthy outdoor life of the boys.

As I have already mentioned, diphtheria can be more safely prevented by the homoeopathic nosode *Diphtherinum*, given in single doses in a high potency. This would not have any serious after effects and would not upset a child's health at all, as immunization so frequently does.

Even if diphtheria broke out, it can be rapidly and easily cured by homoeopathic medication without giving anti-toxin.

Reaction		Length of protection	Remarks
Child	Adult		
Nil or very slight	(See Remarks)	Probably for life	More necessary in children of 1 to 15 than in adults. The whooping cough vaccine can be combined with this, in which case, however, the treatment takes a somewhat longer time

I am now treading on even more dangerous ground.

In one of the homoeopathic hospitals as soon as diphtheria was diagnosed after bacteriological examination, the patients were given the appropriate, indicated medicine, whichever worked out, it is not always the same medicine; and then sent to the Fever Hospital, as there is no isolation ward in the homoeopathic hospital. Several times the medical officer rang up the homoeopathic house surgeon to inform him that there was no diphtheria found on further bacteriological examination, that the cases were on the mend, and surely a mistake had been made at the homoeopathic hospital. On being shown the original slides, he had to acknowledge that the diagnosis was correct and he could not make out what happened afterwards.

A friend of mine reminded me of a case I had seen some ten years ago which I had forgotten. A child who was seen at the clinic with definite signs of diphtheria of the throat, confirmed by bacteriological examinations, was given a dose of *Phytolacca cm* by me, previously to sending her to the Isolation hospital. She was sent home again after four or five days with the report that no diphtheria was found at the hospital. The child was perfectly well.

There are a certain number of homoeopathic physicians who have not sufficient faith in their drugs, but who give doses of injections of anti-toxin, either with or without the homoeopathic medicine. Anti-toxin is absolutely necessary to cure a case of diphtheria they say. I want to know why? If we work according to the law that like cures like, and believe in it, surely diphtheria is not a disease outside and above the law?

There are many remedies which can cure diphtheria and have cured it at the hands of doctors in Switzerland, France, America, England, etc.

One remedy specially has produced certain poisoning effects which are almost identical with diphtheria. This is Cyanide of Mercury, and as Dr. Clarke says: One case of poisoning by Mercury cyanide was actually treated for diphtheria by the attending doctors, before the causal agent was discovered. You get fainting, collapse, trembling with feebleness and nausea and general icy coldness of body with greyish-white membranes inside mouth, cheeks and on tonsils. As this Cyanide of Mercury produces a condition similar to diphtheria, it should cure it, if you get these symptoms in diphtheria. In fact, it is so similar to diphtheria that it should be a prophylactic to this disease, and I believe it has been used as a preventive by some doctors with excellent results, that is in single doses of the 30th potency. I have never tried it myself, but if ever I was faced with a diphtheria epidemic, I should give *Mercurius cyanatus* 30 in some cases and *Diptherinum* 200 or higher in other cases and compare the two results. I guarantee my results would be better than inoculation with the immunizing toxoids that are being advised everywhere.

Dr. Charette in his book, *Practical Materia Medica*, which I am sorry to say has not been translated yet, as far as I know, into English, mentions four cases of severest diphtheria which were cured by Cyanide of Mercury within 2-3 days; the membranes and the high temperature usually disappearing within 40-48 hours. The medicine has to be given dissolved in a tumbler of water and teaspoonful doses taken every quarter hour, until improvement sets in.

Dr. Charette also mentions how one child, after being given a dose of anti-toxin, was extremely ill for three weeks with suppression of urine, violent pains, wasting and extreme weakness, and her brother who was given a prophylactic dose of anti-toxin died within a few minutes of the injection! Moreover, the attending doctor consoled the sorrowing parents by exclaiming 'that the serum had killed many patients and would kill many more'. And Dr. Charette says that the Cyanide of Mercury has a favourable action on diphtheria without any of the inconveniences of the anti-toxin.

Dr. Nash, of America, found *Apis* as the chief healing agent in some epidemics. It is the simillimum for diphtheria cases where this disease comes on exceedingly rapidly and violently, the whole throat filling up with an oedematous swelling, the uvula hanging down like a transparent sac filled with water. The condition is painless until far advanced and the patient is in danger of suffocation by closure of throat and larynx; or sometimes there may be stinging burning pains like bee stings, which are improved by cold applications, and the breathing of course is extremely difficult and noisy. In these cases allopathically the only thing to do is to perform a tracheotomy to prevent suffocation. And yet Dr. Nash cured this case without an operation with *Apis* and says that during that epidemic not one case who took this remedy died, and yet over 40 cases had died of it in that town at that time before *Apis* was given.

Do you see how different an *Apis* case is from a Cyanide of Mercury case?

Then there is *Kali bichromicum, Lycopodium, Lachesis, Lac caninum* and other Mercury Salts — such as *Mercurius protoiodide* and *Mercurius biniodide*, and last but not least, *Phytolacca*; they each, one and all, have their separate and distinctive symptoms and will, if their particular symptoms are found in a case of diphtheria, cure that case within 40-48 hours without any attendant inconveniences and complications such as post-diphtheritic paralysis, heart weakness, muscular rheumatism of the extremities and general enfeeblement — which last is the almost invariable effect of the anti-toxin treatment on top of the original infection, which already has a weakening effect on the heart muscle.

Believe me there is no need for alarmist actions, no need for compulsory inoculations, which will only lead to a deterioration of the health of the victims, which may last for years.

Then there is our nosode, *Diphtherinum*, which I have used only once as a prophylactic in a diphtheria contact. I gave *Dip. cm*, one dose and the disease did not develop; this might have been coincidence, of course. I have used it several times as opportunity offered in post-diphtheritic cases.

A little while ago a girl of 13 was troubled with a constant thick catarrh of the nose with crust formation and painful cracks at the entrance of the nose. These cracks bled and wept for weeks. I tried various remedies:.*Kali bichromicum*, and *Thuja*. Then I discovered this child had been troubled with this off and on practically all through the years ever since a diphtheria attack some years ago. On this information I gave one dose of *Diphtherinum cm*: prompt recovery and no return for ten months. I then lost sight of her. Her brother, slightly younger, presented the same symptoms, and I gave him *Dip. cm* with the same happy results.

Some two years ago I saw a mother who had been extremely deaf with internal ear deafness for nearly 20 years ever since an attack of diphtheria, at the age of ten. *Dip. cm* at intervals of three months, whenever she presented herself, markedly improved her hearing, she could hear and follow ordinary conversation with comparative ease which she had not been able to do for years.

Several months ago I saw a woman in the middle twenties, who became almost stone deaf after diphtheria at the age of 7, and went to a school for the physically handicapped until she was 16 years old. One had to bawl and shout at her and even then she had to refer to her sister who had discovered some patent way of communicating with her. She would not go anywhere without her sister for this reason.

I persuaded her to take a dose of *Dip. cm*, hoping for the best. Four weeks later she came again, minus her sister this time, with her child, aged 2. I spoke to her in my ordinary tone of voice, not remembering her deafness at first and she understood perfectly well and answered correctly. Suddenly I noticed at the top of the case-paper: mother very deaf. I asked her then, had she noticed how much better she could hear and she smilingly agreed, though, being somewhat slow in the uptake, she had not connected it with my powder. I repeated the dose and found deafness improved still more, indeed it had almost gone three months later.

Something great is achieved when hearing is restored so that you can hear the human voice and are able to listen to music and hear the singing of the birds! A deaf person is more shut off from human intercourse than a blind one, and becomes easily cantankerous and suspicious.

It is worth while to go back to the original cause of the deafness, whatever it may be. Deafness comes on after several of the infectious diseases: after measles and influenza, after small-pox, and after meningitis. Remember the respective nosode, give an occasional dose and more than likely an improvement will set in even after such a long period as 20 years. I have proved it. Remember also suppressed skin diseases; *Mezereum* in a case of total deafness after suppression of eczema of the head in infancy brought out the skin trouble again for a short time and cured the deafness. This was related by the late Dr. Dunham in one of his books.

There is much hidden power in our remedies, not to forget our remedies made from disease products, the so-called nosodes, and such chronic suffering, diseases of long standing, could be cleared up if more use were made of them, in unit doses spaced and only repeated at 2- 3- or 4-weekly intervals, or whenever a slipping-back in the patient's condition is noticed.

CHAPTER TWENTY-TWO

ENURESIS OR BED-WETTING

This is a problem ever to the fore where there are children. It has been discussed for years in the medical press with very little result. I carefully followed the advice given in the orthodox professional papers for many months and was sadly disappointed, it seemed to me that other doctors were up a blind alley as well. Psychological treatment is advised; maybe it does good, maybe it does not.

It is true that habit and training from the earliest days of babyhood will make a clean child. You can train a baby to be clean and dry when it is barely eight weeks old, if you persevere and hold it out regularly before and after feeds. It soon learns what is expected of it, after making the appropriate hissing noises with your lips, it empties the bladder and the mother or nurse is saved a great deal of work.

There are periods in a child's life when, in spite of regular training in good habits, it forgets itself; teething irritation may cause an occasional lapse for a few days. Some children may even in their second and third years, in a mood of rebellion and exhibitionism in order to draw the attention of the adults to themselves, refuse to use the appropriate vessel at the appointed times and wait until mother's back is turned to do the necessary. A few well applied smacks to the buttocks soon cures their naughty tricks, in spite of the modern teaching of soft handling of the growing child. The rod judiciously applied in the early days is of immense value in character formation.

I have known children in respectable working class families and even, I must confess to my grief, professional households who should know better, where no attempts were made to train the children in cleanliness and where wet beds were the rule rather than the exception with boys and girls at the age of 4 and 5. The mothers seemed helpless and would rather put up with this inconvenience than remonstrate with the offenders. Again and again I have found that a short period away from home with an understanding grown-up person, who knew how to deal with children, would cure the bed-wetting in a short period of one or two weeks. The child would be held out regularly in the day time, would be made to empty the bladder on going to bed and habitually made to get up every two hours until 11 p.m., and a dry bed was the consequence of just this little extra trouble taken.

There is no fear of a child losing too much sleep if it is got up regularly for this purpose every night; it just drops to sleep again, the moment it is lifted back to bed.

Bed-wetting I am afraid is therefore often the parents' fault in the first instance. A nervous older child may wet the bed in periods of stress, if it is away from home in strange surroundings, or if it is afraid of getting out of bed in the dark. A small nightlight for a period will help to cure this bad habit. I know one boy of 10 who regularly wetted the bed because he was made to use the outside lavatory, and he was afraid of the dark and the loneliness. When the family moved into another house where the lavatory was on the same landing inside the house, the wet beds ceased.

Frequently bed-wetting is caused, too, by a cold bed. The matron of a large well-known boys' preparatory school told me that nearly 50 per cent of the little boys of this school had frequent lapses in their first few months at school. She cured them by placing the beds of these respective boys close to the radiators, and if necessary putting hot bottles in the beds as well. There were practically no failures to report.

These are just a few simple rules which should be tried first to break this unpleasant habit. They do not work in all cases; medical treatment may be necessary as well. I had no success with the old school treatment with ever increasing doses of tincture of belladonna and endocrine gland treatment. I gave them a good trial. Then I applied my knowledge of homoeopathy and I had a very good reputation in the local schools near the dispensary of being able to cure nocturnal enuresis, or bed-wetting, almost at once.

A girl, aged 11, was sent to me by a school doctor on February 25th, 1941, for debility, anaemia and bed-wetting, with which she had been troubled since infancy. The mother was distinctly grouchy and irritable at being sent to yet another place for treatment: 'nobody could cure the girl' she stated, 'why worry, she might grow out of it when she was fourteen.'

She was a small, thin girl, under-sized, with a cowed look, very timid and shy, bad colour, wept easily when spoken to sharply, always tired in the evenings, hated fat food; weight 4 stone 9 lb. 10 oz. Wetted the bed often twice in the night. The urine smelt strongly of ammonia; no history of tuberculosis in the family.

Pulsatilla 30 every night and morning prescribed.

4.3.41 — No wet beds for five nights during this week. The child was duly praised. Always encourage such a child, ask how many nights the bed was dry; not how many times it was wet. Repeat *Puls.* 30 night and morning.

11.3.41. — Weight 4 st. 11 lb. 2 oz. Five dry nights this week. Gained 1½ lb. in a fortnight. Repeat *Puls.* as before.

18.3.41. — Left-sided follicular tonsillitis; very liable to get sore throats — return of an old symptom, which is very common with homoeopathic treatment. The tonsil looked purple, tongue dirty, thickly coated at the base; *in spite of the acute inflammatory condition of the throat there was only one wet bed during the week*. Enlarged tonsils are often said to cause wet beds.

Phytolacca 30, three times daily for three days.

She had lost 4 ozs. in weight which is not surprising.

1.4.41. — Much better colour, not so yellow, still slight enuresis. *Puls.* 30 t.d.s.

She did not turn up for the next three weeks, until April 22nd. — Weight had gone down to 4 st. 10 lb. 12 oz.; five dry nights.

Unit dose of *Sulphur* 30.

April 29th. — No enuresis this week at all. Weight 4 st. 12 lb. 7 oz. A gain of over 1½ lb. in a week; eating well.

May 6th. – No bed-wetting again. Weight 4 st. 12 lb. 12 oz.; always hungry and is enjoying her food.

Mother met me and her whole face was one smile from end to end; said 'she had been attending two different hospitals for years and they had never done any good, and she had received benefit the moment she entered the clinic and now just look at the difference!' Very diffidently she offered me through the nurse as a personal thank-offering two new laid eggs from her own chickens. A very great gift from a poor woman with a family of seven children! A veritable widow's mite. Naturally I received it in the spirit it was given, with pleasure.

It reminded me of my very first fee I received, when I was still a medical student and I treated and cured rapidly the daughter of the landlord of the house I was staying in, who had a bad whitlow of the thumb. I gave her fomentations and doses of *Hepar sulph.* 3*x*, four hourly. The father was so grateful at my having relieved her pain and cured the finger without a surgical operation that he presented me with, I think it was, half a dozen fresh eggs. It might have been a dozen eggs. It is half a life-time ago and I have forgotten the details.

On May 12th this child was seen again. She had gained another ½ lb. and still no further attacks of enuresis.

Repeat *Sulphur* 30 (unit dose).

In a short ten weeks this child had gained 3½ lb. and had been cured of this habit of hers which had made her life a burden. How easy it was, just a few doses of *Pulsatilla* followed by *Sulphur*, given because she had the *Pulsatilla* temperament, and when *Puls.* did not hold any more, followed up by the great psoric remedy *Sulphur*.

Now *Pulsatilla* does not cure every case of bed-wetting, only if the *Pulsatilla* symptoms are present.

I'll give you another case of *Pulsatilla*. She was a little girl of about two years of age, very backward with her teeth, she had only twelve teeth; a very clean, well-trained child, fat and plump, who suddenly developed enuresis, when the eye teeth were coming through, much to her mother's annoyance. She looked typically *Pulsatilla*, was weepy and whined with the teething. I gave her *Pulsatilla* 6, night and morning; the enuresis stopped at once. She only had it for a couple of weeks. *Pulsatilla* 6 was repeated for another two weeks, then *Pulsatilla* 30, and the teeth came through with a run, without further pain or trouble of any kind, and she continued gaining weight all the time. There had been no return of the bed-wetting.

One of my early attempts of curing bed-wetting was in a young lad, aged 15, who had wet beds every night. However hard he tried, he could not cure himself of it. His mother had not wanted him when he was coming and had taken some strong purgatives and repeated doses of quinine and made herself very ill. The child was born in due course, in spite of it all; but to punish her he was somewhat backward and slightly mentally deficient, could not read, had a defect in his speech.

I remembered that Dr. Burnett had said that *Tuberculinum* or *Bacillinum* had cured well nigh on 90 per cent of cases of enuresis in his hands; so I thought that is good enough for me, here goes, I'll follow suit. *Tuberculinum* 30 in weekly doses and later *Tuberculinum m.* were faithfully taken for weeks and the doses were repeated whenever there was a recurrence of the habit.

At once there was great improvement, only one or two wet beds a week and two or three weeks none at all and then only an occasional lapse. After three months a complete cure. With all his mental powers improved, his speech became clearer, and he became much more intelligent. He managed to get into the tailoring trade and became a porter and did very well. All this happened in 1916. I heard from him about a year ago, when he wrote to me from a sanatorium for tuberculosis, reporting that he had developed consumption in spite of leading an out-of-door life as an outside porter delivering parcels to clients. The tendency to tuberculosis was there, and developed later in life. If would not have developed if he had had consecutive homoeopathic treatment; only he left the neighbourhood and I had not seen him for 18 years.

I have found Dr. Burnett to be right. Many cases of bed-wetting have been cured by me since with *Tuberculinum*, even though there is no history of tuberculosis available. Where there is a definite history of consumption, of course *Tuberculinum* must be strongly considered.

A girl of 11 or 12 suddenly developed the habit of bed-wetting while her mother was in hospital and she was staying with friends. There was consumption in the family, so I gave her *Tuberculinum* 30, weekly doses. After a couple of weeks, she was given nightly doses of *Tuberculinum* 30 with an immediate improvement. There was no further trouble, much to the mother's joy.

I could fill a book with the number of cases of enuresis I have cured with *Tuberculinum*, only it would be wearisome — it would be just a repetition.

Sulphur is a very good remedy if there are *Sulphur* symptoms present, or even if there are no other symptoms except just that the wetting is due to a bad habit. *Sulphur* is such a grand psoric remedy that it cures the bad points in the child's family history, and the habit disappears.

If bed-wetting comes on after an acute infectious disease, it can be cured rapidly, almost invariably, with a dose of the respective nosode.

A child of 9 years had enuresis for five or six years, ever since an attack of scarlet fever. *Scarlatinum* 200, weekly doses, cleared up this habit in two weeks.

Another boy had developed bed-wetting after a severe attack of measles, had constant wet beds for six months. Weekly doses of *Morbillinum* 30 and later *Morbillinum* 100 cured the condition in four weeks and made him put on 3 lb. in weight in a month.

There are other remedies which may be required. There was a little boy, aged 9 or 10, with whom I had great difficulties in tracing the right remedy. Eventually I discovered he was afraid of the dark, he was afraid of being alone, he even used to cling to his younger brother, aged 5, for protection in the dark going up to the bedroom, he was nervous of everything, thunder and lightning as well. *Phos.* 30

in repeated doses cured him for months; then he was evacuated and sent to the country. Promptly the bad habit recurred, the billeting officer, a very efficient, bullying type of a lady, dragged him from one doctor to another and he was scolded and punished and psycho-analysed, all to no effect. Eventually his mother came to me and with tears in her eyes implored me to help her. The boy was brought back and a few doses of *Phosphorus* 30 completely cured him again in a week. I then advised the mother to betake herself and her two boys to the country to the same billet, stocked her with *Phos.* 30 and told her to write when and if the trouble returned. That was four months ago. I have had no news so far.

Another boy, about 10 years old, was very retiring, always stayed indoors, always afraid of other children, always worrying about the school, woke up in the night shouting about the school. Very tired in the early afternoon. *Lycopodium* 30 in weekly doses did the trick here.

Bed-wetting is a trouble which can be treated successfully and rapidly with homoeopathic remedies provided you know your remedies. There are no specific drugs for this unpleasant anti-social complaint, study each individual case, take the history, and almost invariably the cure is rapid, sometimes almost startlingly so.

CHAPTER TWENTY-THREE

EAR DISCHARGE

A running ear, as it is colloquially called, is a very unpleasant complaint, and the sufferer is a nuisance not only to himself but also to his neighbours from the disgusting odour which is associated with this trouble.

Unfortunately for the patient as well as for his relatives and friends, this complaint is extremely difficult to deal with. It usually persists for years and years; and orthodox medicine has very little to offer in the matter of a permanent cure.

It seems to run in families; several members are frequently affected with it. And in elementary schools the incidence of discharging ears is high, which makes one suspect that wrong feeding, not underfeeding, is at the bottom of it. Devitalized and especially demineralised foods are one of the causes, I am sure. The diet in the working-class homes consists of tea, condensed milk, white bread, jam and margarine, foreign chilled or frozen meat, and tinned fruit. Very little fresh fruit and very little fresh vegetables are consumed; moreover, these are deprived of their mineral contents by being swamped in an excess of water and further alkalinised with bicarbonate of soda, which is said to retain the green colour of the vegetables and does this by throwing out more of the minerals into the water, which all goes down the drain after being boiled. The results we see every day: ill health, constipation, no resistance to infection of any kind, it may be colds or chills or bronchitis or sore throats which lead to septic infection of the ear. Measles, scarlet fever and diphtheria are also common causes of septic throats, and thus are forerunners of septic ear infections.

The orthodox treatment for running ears is mainly surgical: removal of the septic tonsils and adenoids and, if this does not work, an operation on the mastoid bone. This is said to finish the trouble; how often, alas! this proves wrong. With every fresh chill there is a return of the running ear; a reinfection occurs in the tonsils or tonsilar area and it travels up the Eustachian tube into the ear. Does this not prove to those of us who can see further that the cause of this recurrent trouble is not the ubiquitous bacillus or coccus, but the individual in question whose constitution presents a suitable soil for the bacteria to thrive on. And what is needed is not a surgical operation or a series of operations, but the building up of the constitution of the child. Not by means of so-called tonics or gallons of cod-liver oil and malt or Parrish's food, but the reconditioning of the structure of the human body by the indicated homoeopathic remedy. *Homoeopathic, not because it is given in small doses, but because the remedy is similar to the symptoms presented by the individual.* There are no specific remedies for running ears; one person may be cured by one remedy and the next by a totally different one. Study each person as he or she comes along, and you will find that running ears no longer remain chronic, they dry up and in time the patient will stand up to a chill; and the ear will not become reinfected. This may take time, but it is promising work, and well worth while.

I have seen and treated hundreds of cases of discharging ears at my dispensary, and the same children used to attend year after year from the time they were infected, usually after measles or scarlet fever, right until they left school: five, six, seven or eight years in many cases. They had their tonsils out, their adenoids were removed, their ear-drums were incised and, lastly, the mastoid bone was operated on.

I have known both mastoids being done, not only once, but two or three times. It was disheartening work, until I started to apply my homoeopathic knowledge to these cases; and then we suddenly saw the children's ears clear up in a great many cases.

Unfortunately elementary school children are so much inspected now that before a case is completely cured or even after the ear is no longer discharging, the child is ordered to hospital for a mastoid operation, and I have seen pitiful examples of children whose ears were perfectly dry and no longer discharging being sent to hospital for surgical treatment, and come out after months and months of in-patient treatment, with hideous scars and sometimes completely deaf and, in spite of it all, the ears were again discharging. Some were successful, I agree, but a fair percentage of mastoid operations were anything but successful; they still had to carry on with zinc ionisation, just as before the operation. One girl I recall had two mastoid operations, then as the wound would not heal up and there was a large raw area, she was taken in again and the ear was skin-grafted. It still went on discharging, and there was a sinus two inches long with a small opening just big enough to admit a probe going down to the base of the abscess in the mastoid. This girl was 12 years of age, very backward, very quiet and retiring, squashed and sat upon by everybody, white and transparent and anaemic, always looked tired and weary and listless, cried easily when spoken to, yet quietly obstinate and would not respond to any kindness.

This mental make-up, with the long history of septic infection of the ear and chronic abscess, made one think of *Silica*; and *Silica* 30 was given whenever required, at first weekly and after a while monthly. The effect on the sinus was quite remarkable. The offensive odour went, the discharge instead of being thick and purulent became thin like clear serum and then it dried up and the ear healed over, the opening leading to the bone closed up. And the girl herself brightened up, became cheerful and happy, talked and chattered, got on better at school, and her cheeks filled out. She attended off and on and was kept under observation for two years, until she left school, and there was no return of her running ears for the last eighteen months after seven long years of treatment for otorrhoea. A few doses of *Silica* did the trick. At the time we were all very interested in this case, as she had been treated for many years for the same complaint. It gave me heart to try and treat other ear cases with the appropriate medicine, and with experience one has added to the ever-lengthening list of cured cases.

A child aged 9 turned up on November 12th, 1940, with a history of a right-sided mastoid operation after the ear had been running for two years. The ear was in a pitiable state. One knew she was near because of the penetrating foul odour; the lobe of the ear was raw, inflamed and blistered, where the acrid discharge had run over; this blistering was all round the opening of the ear. A thorough mess. The ear was dried out and powdered whenever she came in; she was rather irregular in attendance and she was given a dose of *Tellurium* 6 every two or three days. On November 26th the ear discharge had dried up, the cracks and blistering of the lobe of the ear had healed up, and there was, of course, no more smell from the ear. Seen on December 10th, the child still looks white and pasty, but the ear remains dry, the opening in the drum has closed up. She will require further treatment in order to prevent a reinfection; but to dry up a chronic ear discharge in two weeks is wonderful. *Tellurium* is a remedy to be thought of in otorrhoea, when you get this terrible penetrating odour like fish brine from the ear with reddening and inflammation of the skin near it.

The discharge is foetid, stained with blood, thin and watery serum and occasionally purulent, but the odour is *the* characteristic, and the bluish, reddish discolouration of the skin with excoriation and blistering. Such a discharge with these characteristics is apt to come on after scarlet fever, and is cured with *Tellurium*. I have only used it in the 6th potency, and it has served me well again and again.

Ear discharges vary a great deal: for example, *Graphites* has an offensive discharge resembling fish brine like *Tell.*, but the discharge is glutinous and sticky with the consistency and colour of honey and there is no blistering where the discharge touches the skin. The *Graphites* child feels the cold, the draught and cold damp weather and the excessive heat. A fat pale child with a waxy appearance of the face, the skin chaps and cracks easily everywhere, is harsh and dry, and he has an aversion to eating meat and — which is peculiar — an aversion to eating sweets, and with it is inclined to be constipated. It is an impudent child, who laughs at being scolded and reprimanded, teasing and bold and forward. Such a child with otorrhoea will be cured by *Graphites* in a short time.

I recall a boy who first started having earache at the age of nine months, frequent attacks of bronchitis and severe tonsillitis and septic glands of the neck. On February 7th, 1935, when three years old, both drums were incised for earache.

In March, 1935, tonsils were removed, as they were septic. They were slow in healing after the operation. In September, 1935, another attack of severe earache. In spite of months and months on Parrish's food he remained pale and anaemic, his nose was obstructed and he was a mouth-breather. On January 10th, 1936, his adenoids were removed; recurrent attacks of tonsillitis followed; festering sores on body all through 1936 and 1937.

On February 10th, 1938, acute inflammation of the right ear following an attack of tonsillitis. The drum was incised twice during February, 1938. Right mastoid operation performed early in March, 1938. He looked wretched and miserable after all this, very nervous and timid, restless, afraid of the dark and of being alone, in some ways very precocious. He was just 6 years old, the face was very white and pallid, lips were red. The ear was still discharging freely, though he had the operation nearly three weeks previously; in desperation I gave *Bacillus Gaertner* 30 on March 21st, 1938. He had *Lycopodium, Strept.* and *Pulsatilla* repeatedly before, during the previous three years, with only temporary relief.

On April 4th, 1938, ear discharge clearing up, eating well, face much better colour, not nearly so nervous. *Gaertner* 30.

April 11th. Repeat; colour shows great improvement.

May 16th, 1938. Very active and bright, not so shy. Still a sinus in the ear. Repeat *Gaertner* 30.

June 13th, 1938. Skin grafting to be done, as sinus not yet closed. *Silica* 30.

Silica is a near relative to *Gaertner bacillus* and as the ear wound was so long in healing up, a dose of *Silica* seemed to be indicated.

On July 4th, 1938. Skin grafting done, scar looks healthy.

Gaertner 30 given, which was repeated on four occasions until July, 1939, when the child was last seen. He then looked fit and well, a sturdy chap, and had not had a recurrence of his ear trouble. The improvement set in as soon as the *Gaertner bacillus* was given early in 1938.

The family has moved away, so one does not know what happened to him; certainly while he was under the action of this bowel nosode, he flourished and made great strides.

I have since found that the *Gaertner* nosode does well in septic conditions, if the child is thin and flabby and mentally restless and precocious, and has nervous fears — of darkness and solitude.

His younger brother started to go the same way, became very anaemic and pale, with red lips; had earache. So I put him on *Gaertner* 30. In six weeks he gained 1½ lb. and had two teeth as well, his colour became fresh and rosy. He walked at twelve months, when he weighed 24¾ lb., with six teeth. He was well over weight, sturdy and healthy, with no signs of rickets, all firm muscle, no superfluous fat.

At fourteen months an attack of earache was aborted with a dose of *Gaertner* 30. Every two or three months he had another dose of *Gaertner* and had no further attacks of tonsillitis and only mild attacks of earache with each new tooth until July, 1939, when at the age of 2 years he weighed 29½ lb., had nineteen teeth and was in good condition all round. He started to go like his brother, with tonsillitis and earache; but the tendency was stopped with the appropriate medicine.

Then unfortunately they left London, and nothing further has been heard of the family.

Another case who responded rapidly to *Bacillus Gaertner* comes to my mind.

A boy about eight months old with flabby muscles and pallid complexion developed profuse ear discharge. He had five teeth, was able to stand and walk round chairs, very forward and precocious and weighed 16½ lb. After the first dose of *Gaertner* 30 the ear discharge improved within a week; a fortnight later the perforation of the drum had healed over and there was no further discharge from the ear. The scalp was sweating slightly during sleep, and *Silica* 30, a close relation of *Gaertner*, was then given, which hastened the eruption of his teeth so that a month later he had ten teeth, five new teeth in a month, and gained ¾ lb. in weight as well; which is also unusual. A child struggling with teeth as a rule remains stationary or loses weight. But I find children under homoeopathic treatment get their teeth easily, do not disturb their parents at night and usually put on weight as well. The teeth just come through without any trouble.

All this happened four months ago. He is now fourteen months old, has got sixteen teeth, weighs 20 lb., walks well and, though small-boned, is active and lively, and shows no further signs of any ear trouble, though my experience tells me that once a child gets a running ear with a tooth it recurs with every new tooth. But the homoeopathic medicine properly applied cuts right across the vicious circle and builds up the child at the same time.

Remember, the *Gaertner* child or the child who requires *Gaertner* is in appearance like *Silica*, pale, thin, flabby, but is more precocious and has the nervous fears of *Phosphorus*. Sometimes you have to give the one, sometimes the other, after *Gaertner*.

On August 19th, 1940, a three-months-old baby was seen with a profusely running left ear. Weight 13½ lb. The mother had a sore throat at the same time; the infection came from her, the child's throat was swollen as well and the inflammation had travelled up to the middle ear and had made an opening through the drum. As the discharge was clear and honey-like, *Graphites* 30 was prescribed; but on August 26th the discharge was worse, more offensive, more purulent, and the left lobe of the ear was red and inflamed on the outside. Something more was required, and as there was sepsis and a rash on the ear, I argued, it must be a streptococcal infection; throats which are intensely red frequently are due to the streptococcus, and this streptococcus nearly always produces an erythema of the skin, as you see in erysipelas and in scarlet fever.

So I gave *Streptococcus* 200 in the unit dose on that day and repeated it a week later. Improvement set in a week after and the whole thing cleared up without any bother after the second dose. On October 3rd the child had some perspiration of the scalp. There was a crack above the left ear. So I gave *Silica* 30 one dose and repeated it on October 24th; and on November 7th the crack behind and above the ear had gone; the ear had given no further trouble and the child had put on 3 lb. in ten weeks. Now at seven months he weighs 17¾ lb. and the first tooth is showing.

The remedies made from potentized emulsions of various types of bacilli and cocci work very well, and their symptoms are derived largely from the effects they produce on the suffering individual. The presumably healthy person gets infected with a dose of say streptococcus and produces certain skin, throat and ear symptoms. If you get these symptoms and there are no definite strong indications for a homoeopathic remedy, give a dose or two of the potentized *Streptococcus*; this will antidote the poison, the toxin, and clear the deck for another remedy: it may be *Silica* or *Sulphur* or *Phosphorus* or may be another. The symptoms showing the need for another remedy will show up. So it is with any other bacillus such as *Gaertner* bacillus, etc. There are a number of bacillary nosodes, as they are called, and very pretty work can be done with them in various infections, especially in children's diseases. Dr. Bach first worked them out, and later each bowel nosode was individualized by the Glasgow school of physicians; their mental symptoms were observed, their physical characteristics noted. I for one should not like to be without these potentized coccal and bacillary remedies.

For example, I know a lady of over 60 who had a severe mastoid operation when she was 11 years old. She has had trouble with her ears off and on since; she gets some moisture and traces of blood now and then and the ear wax is excessive at times, and when she gets over-tired her deafness is very marked. She has been treated homoeopathically for years for all her ailments; whenever the deafness troubles her more and the discharge begins to appear, an occasional dose of *Streptococcus* 200 will clean up the ear, the discharge dries up and the deafness improves as well. So the original streptococcal infections can be antidoted even after more than fifty years!

Another lady of nearly 40 had three mastoid operations in her teens, the last when she was 21 years of age. Her left ear is continually giving her trouble. A tremendous lot of dry wax is being formed and some horrible-smelling dry hard masses are continually found in the ear cavity which is huge after the repeated operations, and this offensive cerumen mixed with blood and dead skin has got to be removed in a week or so, or she gets giddy turns from the pressure of this débris on the ear. Occasional doses of *Streptococcus* 200 improve the giddiness and diminish the amount of ear wax; I am wondering whether, by giving a higher potency, one could not stop this excessive formation of cerumen entirely. Anyway, until the *Streptococcus* was given, the trouble in her ear was almost more than she could bear.

Another pretty little case who not only had a chronic ear discharge but several other complications follows.

On February 29th, 1940, a girl of 10 years of age was brought by her granny for running ears. She was a girl big and heavy for her age, who used to be treated at one of the special ear clinics for this discharging ear. She had her tonsils removed when she was 5 years old. The discharging ears dated back to an attack of scarlet fever treated in hospital when she was only six weeks old. Otorrhoea going back to scarlet fever in infancy! – in spite of constant treatment at home by general practitioners, in hospital, operation on the tonsils at the age of 5, an operation for septic glands at another hospital at twelve months, there was no improvement. No wonder the child was nervous and frightened of doctors. I could do nothing with her the first time. The right drum was scarred, the left drum showed a perforation. There was also a severe squint, for which she was wearing glasses. She suffered from bed-wetting which was a nightly occurrence; the poor grandmother had looked after her since she was 5 years old, as the mother had run away from her husband and family.

A nice complicated case! And the puzzle was where to start with treatment. She had had Parrish's food, she had had other tonics, no doubt cod-liver oil and malt, etc., and nothing had done her any good. She only came to get her ear cleaned up, and I started to clean her up from the bottom. First she was given *Scarlatinum, 200* as the trouble began after scarlet fever.

On March 7th, 1940, a week later, I was told more about her. She was very nervous, dull of understanding, said to have no brains, cannot read properly yet, even though she was in her 11th year; is very fond of housework, but refuses to take an interest in her lessons. Her intellect and nervous system had been examined at Maudsley Hospital. She gets very cross and angry and cries when she does not get her own way. She will not stay indoors, but is always out playing in the street. The discharge from the left ear has nearly stopped after one week's treatment! — *Tuberculinum* 30.

March 21st. Left drum: healing perforation; is very stubborn, tells a great many lies, says she has been attending at the centre for her ears, and has not been near us for treatment. Very difficult to examine, cries and whimpers and objects strongly. *Tuberculinum* 30.

March 28th. Right drum of cerumen and dead skin. Very severe squint; nervous and afraid of school. *Lycopod.* 30.

April 4th. Temper much better, attends regularly. Left drum healed completely. *Lycopod.* 30.

April 11th. Twitching and nystagmus of both eyes; backward mentally, can spell but refuses to put letters together into words. *Lycopod.* 30.

April 18th, 1940. Not so nervous and frightened. *Lueticum* 30.

April 25th. Much quieter, used to be most unruly and unmanageable, very restless and fidgety — can sit still now. *Leuticum* 30.

May 2nd, 1940. Slight moisture again from left ear. *Scarlatinum* 200.

May 9th. Left drum perforation drying up and healing again; much better in herself. Quieter, more composed. Has wetted the bed for over five years, no more bed-wetting now since her first attendance at the centre nine weeks ago. 'Almost too good to be true,' her grandmother says. *Scarlatinum* 200.

May 16th. Lazy at school, does not trouble to read. *Sulph.* 30, repeated May 23rd.

May 30th. Left ear perforation healed. Right drum offensive discharge like rancid cheese, very tender to touch; hates having her ear done. *Hepar sulph.* 30.

June 6th. Both drums dry again. Squint much improved, hardly noticeable, eyes almost straight; the twitching of the eyes had disappeared. Very happy now, sings all day, used to be miserable and naughty. No medicine.

July 23rd, 1940. Can sit very still and quiet now. Hardly squints. Ear bled three days ago as nurse was rough with her. I suspect the child played her up and moved at the wrong time. *Hepar sulph.* 30, three times daily.

August 6th. Ears healed, well all round. No offensive smell from ears. *Streptococcus* 200.

September 3rd, 1940. Squint nearly disappeared, only noticeable occasionally. Ears well. Nothing to complain of. A totally different child mentally and physically, since she first came at the end of February, six months previously; even tries to read now!

This girl had running ears, a squint, suffered from bed-wetting, could not read, was mentally backward; in consequence of her disabilities she was unhappy, miserable, contrary and naughty. In a short six months what a difference! Eyes well, ears well, bladder trouble corrected, temper gone. The child looked healthy and blooming.

Yes, one can perform such miracles with Homoeopathy. I have seen many such miserable, unhappy specimens of humanity during the course of many years of medical work at hospitals and dispensary; and I could not touch them until I treated them with Homoeopathy.

In this case still another nosode was used, namely the

nosode derived from scarlet fever. The history was so definite; all the trouble dated back to scarlet fever, and the scarlet fever antidote in a minutest dose started the cure. You will see there are *no* specifics for a running ear, no routine treatment; each case has to be treated on its own merits.

Now for another case, seen for the first time on December 16th, 1940. The child, a very intelligent though under-nourished girl of 6 years of age, had been discharged two weeks previously from a fever hospital after a four months' in-patient treatment for measles followed by scarlet fever. Her right ear was discharging freely, both her eyelids were raw, inflamed and sore with what is commonly called blight, or conjunctivitis; the eyelashes were glued together and encrusted with thick yellow crusts. She was pale, pasty and unhealthy-looking, the haemoglobin content of the red blood corpuscles was only 50 per cent. During the many years of medical practice one has seen hundreds of cases of this ilk who attended the dispensary for months and years even, without the slightest or only very little improvement with the usual local applications for eyes and ears. Some cases were drafted to a residential eye hospital where they stayed frequently for six, twelve, and even eighteen months' treatment. Here they were said to have special nourishment, extra milk, butter, cod-liver oil and malt and vitamins A and D, and with all this extra food it took many months to cure them; and frequently I have known these children to be as bad as ever as soon as they returned to their own homes. What an expense this represents to the ratepayers! A large old country house with beautiful grounds, a large nursing staff, several doctors, given up entirely to the care of poor underfed children suffering from eye diseases. Very laudable indeed; but I claim all this is superfluous, and these children can be cured at home in their ordinary surroundings within a very short time.

My little girl was given a dose of *Morbillinum*, the measles nosode, in the 30th potency; I meant to follow this up, if necessary, with the scarlet fever nosode. The ear was ordered to be cleaned and dried out daily with pledgets of cotton wool; the eyes were washed out with a weak solution of *Euphrasia* and vaseline applied to the eyelashes. Very simple treatment, you say, and not expensive.

She was seen again on December 31st, two weeks later. The mother told me, 'The right ear has stopped discharging, but the left ear is running; the eyes are perfectly all right.' On examination, I found the perforation of the right drum of the ear had healed over and the ear was indeed well. The discharge of the left ear was only wax, and was quickly dealt with. There was no eye trouble at all any more. The *Euphrasia* had cleared up the conjunctivitis, and the eyelashes were minus crusts, and healthy. All this in a fortnight. The child no longer looked pasty and white, there was a bloom on her cheeks. She was given another dose of *Morbillinum* 30 and told to report daily and have her eyes and ears looked at and, if necessary, they were to be treated as before.

I do not expect her to require any further treatment. And when I think of the many children who might have been cured as rapidly during the last twenty years, if I had only known of the *Morbillinum* nosode for eye and ear troubles after measles and *Scarlatinum*, the scarlet fever nosode, for the same trouble following scarlet fever, it makes me sad. And all over the country there are thousands and thousands of cases who should be treated the same way. Much suffering would be saved them.

CHAPTER TWENTY-FOUR

MORBILLINUM (MEASLES SERUM)

Measles is always with us and from being somewhat slightingly spoken of as a complaint safe to be left in the hands of mothers and nannies without medical supervision, it has now been recognized as a potent cause of prolonged invalidism and ill-health in children. More than 13,000 fresh cases of measles have been notified each week during May and June, in England and Wales alone; true the death rate is small, only 10 to 12 cases weekly are certified as having died from it, less than 1 per 1,000. But the after-effects are frequently most serious; chronic recurrent eye affections, such as blepharitis and conjunctivitis, lasting for years, are traceable to measles. Anaemia, weakness, debility and even latent tuberculosis may flare up after it. Frequently one is told that a child has never been well since an attack of measles, and had to take cod-liver oil and malt or an iron tonic for months afterwards, and our convalescent homes are full of cases of weakness and debility after measles or measles plus whooping-cough.

The modern way of treatment of mitigating this is by means of injections of a serum obtained from convalescent cases. At any rate I have come across children who were discharged from the fever hospitals after such inoculations for whom monthly reports were asked for, which had to be sent to the Medical Officer of Health, as to the effects, favourable or otherwise. Modern medicine is slowly groping its way to the truths given out to the world nearly 150 years ago by Hahnemann, that like cures like, only the orthodox *will* give too large doses and thereby produce an aggravation which puts them off the scent therefore and starts them on different treatment.

Our school has used measles serum or nosode, *Morbillinum*, as we call it, for well over fifty years, at any rate the late Dr. Burnett used it in the nineties or even earlier in the last century with good effect; he even cured tumours with it, which he claimed often came on after severe measles. Whether you believe it or not, the tumours did disappear, or a high percentage of them.

Morbillinum is prepared, like any other homoeopathic remedy, diluted according to the 1 in 100 scale, shaken up or succussed at each step, until the desired potency is reached and, like all nosodes, or disease products, should not be given too low, or you might cause a serious aggravation. Even the 6th dilution on the 1 in a 100 scale causes powerful reactions sometimes and it is safer not to give *Morbillinum* or any other nosode below the 30th potency. Some homoeopathic physicians condemn the use of the nosodes, but provided they are given on their proper indications, I find, they do an immense amount of good.

Lately I have come across a number of children who had measles in the late autumn and early winter of last year, and definitely suffered from weakness, loss of weight and anaemia, and in some cases from eye lesions as well. I gladly seized this opportunity of watching the effects of *Morbillinum*, and I must say I was more than agreeably surprised at the results I got.

(1) Peter, aged 1 year 11 months, seen on 9.1.41. Measles in December, 1940, in hospital for two weeks, evidently only a mild case, yet he was fretful and whiny, refused food, wanted to be nursed, 16 teeth, had pharyngitis and tonsillitis and anaemia, very tottery on his feet; no treatment given except cod-liver oil and malt. Seen a month later, on February 10th, conditions unaltered; cervical glands tender and rather larger than before, throat if anything worse; cannot or will not walk at all. Weight 25 lb. 9 oz., thin and flabby – is 2¼ lb. below normal weight. *Morbillinum* 100.

Seen on 3.3.41; put on 18 oz. in three weeks, and produced a new tooth as well, good colour, is happy and bright, laughs and chatters. Rep. *Morb.* 100.

On 24.3.41, lost 10 oz., has got bronchitis, probably due

to sleeping on cold stone floors in the tube shelter; lungs full of scattered rhonchi, moans and wants to be carried; is teething. *Morb.* 100, 1 dose and *Puls.* 6, three times daily for acute condition.

2.4.41. Gained 4 oz., lungs clear, had been suffering from bed-wetting ever since his attack of measles; but no bed-wetting during this last week. *Morb.* 100.

21.4.41. Gained nearly 2 lb. during last three weeks: weight now 28 lb. 4 oz.; no enuresis. Rep. *Morb.* 100.

8.5.41. 20 teeth; weight 28 lb. 14 oz. *Morb.*repeated; a gain of 3¼ lb. in three months since the first dose of *Morbillinum*, and 4 teeth erupted during that period as well.

(2) Girl, seen 23.1.41 − 4 years of age, 5 lb. under weight, very nervous and weepy, cried when examined, left foot is said to hurt her, limps, cannot put foot to the ground properly; nothing found except muscular weakness and tendency to flat feet; glands of the neck are enlarged and tender; anaemic, pallid cheeks; had measles twice; was 9 weeks in hospital lately with measles; discharged two weeks previously. *Puls.* 30 given for general condition and exercises for flat feet ordered.

30.1.41. Gained 4 oz., weight now 31 lb. 7 oz., legs and feet stronger, and left foot hardly painful, much more lively. *Morb.* 100. Convalescence asked for, as mother was very anxious about her.

Seen on 8.5.41, after 12 weeks' convalescence. Weight 33 lb. 9 oz., gained 2 lb., whether due to change of air or *Morbillinum* cannot be determined. Personally, judging from other cases, she would have done even better if she had stayed in London and had regular homoeopathic treatment; the improvement started anyway before she left for the country. Has urticaria now, an old trouble. *Sulph.* 30 given.

(3) Boy, aged 4 years 5 months, seen on 30.12.40. Measles in November, has septic sores in left groin, ankles and right hand, thick nasal catarrh; is under-seized, flabby and thin. Weight 29 lb. 4 oz., in thick winter clothes. *Sulph.* 30.

He gained weight steadily for two months on weekly doses of *Sulph.* 30, until he weighed 31 lb. 2 oz. on 27.2.41; still has sores in left groin and a wart on his right knee. Remembering his history of measles in November, I ordered *Morb.* 100.

13.3.41. Weight 31 lb. 12 oz. Sores in groin, nearly gone; had these since the measles.

10.4.41. Weight 32 lb. 8 oz., eating well. The wart on his knee has disappeared. *Morb.* 100. Weekly doses of *Morbillinum* given since. Weight now, early in June, is 33 lb. Still very much under-weight for his age, but he is of small build, and has small bones. His father and mother are both small and thin. He is extremely well and lively otherwise; has gained 4 lb. since his treatment started, lost his wart and his impetigo.

(4) This child was seen regularly at the clinic until 12.12.40, when he weighed 19 lb. 1 oz. at the age of 14 months and had 16 teeth; had no illnesses, was well formed, though tiny, his muscles were firm, very forward with his teeth, 16 instead of the usual 8. Then his mother trotted off with him to Cambridgeshire, where he developed measles; we did not see him again until 6.2.41, when his weight was 18 lb. 3 oz., a loss of 1½ lb., is flabby and pale, has bronchitis as well. *Morb.* 100.

13.2.41. A week later. Weight 18 lb. 15 oz., cough gone entirely, gained 12 oz. *Morb.* 100.

20.2.41. Weight 20 lb. 2 oz., nearly 2 lb. gained in 2 weeks. *Morb.* 100.

20.3.41. Weight 21 lb. *Morb.* 100.

He got further doses of *Morbillinum* on April 17th, 24th, May 1st, 22nd, and again on June 12th. His weight up to date is 22 lb. 9 oz.; his last 4 teeth have come through as well without any trouble. A gain of 4¼ lb. in 4 months. Now that all his teeth are through, I expect him to romp ahead and gain weight rapidly.

(5) Iris, aged 10½ months; weight 16 lb. 5 oz., has 6 teeth.

Seen on 10.2.41, cannot sit up yet, falls sideways when placed on her mother's lap, muscles flabby and soft, not been well since measles in November, stools alternately loose and constipated, thick nasal catarrh. *Morb.* 100.

10.3.41, a month later. Weight 18 lb. 12 oz. Sitting up now, tries to stand against chair, pulls herself up, no nasal catarrh, no emulsion or cod liver oil and malt given, even though ordered, so gain in weight due to medicine.

17.3.41. 2 more teeth through without any fuss. Weight 19 lb. 2 oz., bowels normal, standing up by herself. A gain of nearly 3 lb. and 2 teeth in one month on 2 doses of *Morbillinum*.

(6) Jean, aged 5½ years. Seen on 9.1.41. Weight 40 lb. 8 oz., nearly 4 lb. underweight, not well since measles in December, looks pale and is thin and flabby, *Morb.* 100.

23.1.41. Weight 41 lb., looking better.

6.2.41. Weight 41 lb. 10 oz. Appetite good.

27.2.41. Weight 42 lb. 8 oz. *Morb.* 100.

10.3.41. Weight 42 lb. 15 oz. Gained 2½ lb. since 9.1.41 in 2 months. *Morb.* 100. Very well and lively.

The usual gain in weight in children of this age is 1 lb. in 3 months.

(7) Ernest, aged 15 months, seen on 13.2.41. Weight 22 lb. 5 oz., had measles early in January, home from hospital just a week; has nasal catarrh, lungs full of catarrhal sounds, 12 teeth. *Morb.* 100.

24.2.41. Weight 23 lb. 4 oz., gain of a lb. in 11 days, doing well. *Morb.* 100.

13.3.41. Weight 23 lb. 15 oz., looks well.

24.3.41. Weight 24 lb. 6 oz. *Morb.* 100.

Gained 2 lb. in 6 weeks on 2 doses of the measles nosode. Nasal catarrh disappeared during the first week of treatment.

(8) Boy, aged 5½ years, seen on 25.2.41. Weight 39 lb. 6 oz. Not well since measles in December; has recurrent attacks of vomiting every 2 weeks since he was 15 months

old. Glands of neck enlarged and tender to touch. *Morb.* 100.

4.3.41. Gained ¼ lb. Seems brighter. *Morb.* 30.

11.3.41. Glands almost gone, better colour, not so white. *Morb.* 30.

18.3.41. No attacks of vomiting since coming here. *Morb.* 30.

1.4.41. Much improved. *Morb.* 30.

29.4.41. Weight 40 lb. 6 oz., gained 1 lb. in 2 months. *Morb.* 30.

Attack of vomiting during week, the first for two months instead of the usual two weekly periodicity.

13.5.41. Tonsillitis. Is said to fret after baby who died last year. *Ignatia* 30 night and morning.

10.6.41. Tonsillitis cleared up within a few days; glands gone; no gain in weight; further constitutional treatment will be necessary — remembering the history of repeated periodic vomiting previous to attack of measles — but he looks well, has a clear skin, pink cheeks and bright eyes, very lively and active.

Now for some cases of eye inflammations dating back to measles.

(9) June K., aged 10, seen 5.9.40, has had inflammation of the eyes since an attack of measles at the age of 5 or 6. Was at Swanley convalescent home for 2 years for her eyes, came back to her parents in August, 1939, and attended an Eye Hospital in this neighbourhood for a while last year. Present condition: corneal opacity of the right eye, stye left lower eyelid, pallid, almost waxy look. Weight 3 st. 11 lb. 8 oz. *Euphrasia* lotion locally for eye. *Morb.* 30.

12.9.40. Eye much better already. Weight 3 st. 11 lb. 14 oz., septic pimple below lid. Rep. *Euphrasia* locally and *Morb.* 30.

24.9.40. Stye gone. Corneal opacity not so noticeable. General appearance: colour much improved. *Morb.* 30.

Child has been lost sight of; she went hopping at the end of September and has not returned to London; but she was a different child after just 3 weeks' treatment.

(10) June W., aged 5½ years. Seen on 17.12.40, just discharged from hospital after three months' stay. Had scarlet fever and contracted measles there; now, 2 weeks home; right ear is discharging, perforation of drum seen, and very offensive discharge; both eyes inflamed, blepharitis and conjunctivitis; wears glasses for squint, is said to be long sighted. *Morb.* 30, *Euphrasia* lotion for eyes; right ear is wiped out daily.

31.12.40. Right ear, perforation healed, no discharge; blepharitis and conjunctivitis nearly cleared up; right ear lobe cracked. Continue local eye treatment as before; *Calendula* ointment for ear. *Morb.* 30.

7.1.41. Nasal catarrh due to lying on cold stone floor in shelter. *Morb.* 30.

14.1.41. Right ear perforation healed, cracked ear dry; squint not so marked.

21.1.41. Right ear discharging slightly again; spends nights in draughty tube station, sleeping on the stone floor; pharyngitis and tonsillitis; slight blepharitis. *Morb.* 30.

28.1.41. Sores round right ear, discharge drying up, eyes nearly well.

4.2.41. Right ear perforation healed again, eyes well. *Morb.* 30. Looking very well; has lost her worried look; is very bright and cheerful.

13.5.41. Seen again after 3 months. Child very well, no return of eye and ear trouble; very good colour. This child lost her ear discharge after only 2 weeks' treatment, though her mother told me that the hospital kept her for many weeks because of this discharge. The slight relapse due to a fresh throat infection also cleared up quickly. Everybody remarked on the general improvement all round; she was the talk of the neighbourhood because she looked so different, after such a short time. Unfortunately she was treated very unkindly by her mother, who talked openly in front of her of what a nuisance she was and that she wanted to get rid of her; then she sent her away through the school authorities in February, after her eyes and ear had cleared up, and only brought her back for a few days in May. Such a pity. She was an extraordinarily intelligent and observant child, so chatty and she made many original remarks to the sister who treated her and appeared to be the leader of older children even in the street.

(11) Charles, aged 13. 28.1.41. Conjunctivitis and blepharitis off and on for years; has been treated for these complaints for at least 4 years at the clinic. *Euphrasia* lotion, *Sulph.* 30.

11.2.41. Eyes improving; twitching of face and shoulders. *Phos.* 30 prescribed for nervous condition; nervous of thunderstorms and darkness. *Euphrasia* lotion for eyes.

18.2.41. Twitching better; eyes sticky of a morning; repeat *Phos.* and *Euphrasia* locally.

25.2.41. History of measles as a baby. *Morb.* 30.

4.3.41. Ulcer on right conjunctiva (aggravation?). Repeat *Euphrasia* and *Morbillinum* 30 daily. Why I prescribed the *Morbillinum* daily the notes do not reveal.

11.3.41. Ulcer right eye cleared up, no more blepharitis; twitching gone.

Seen beginning of May in the street, looks very well. When he attended the dispensary on previous occasions, the local treatment had to be given for usually anything from 4 to 6 months; this time the eyes got well in 2 months, in fact 2 weeks after the *Morbillinum* was first given, the eyes were cured.

(12) Boy. Seen 3.9.40, 11 years old, severe bilateral conjunctivitis and blepharitis since measles 5 years previously. Was at Swanley Eye Hospital as an in-patient for 3 months, 2 years ago. *Morb.* 30, and *Euphrasia* lotion.

24.9.40. Eyes cleared up after only 3 weeks' treatment.

(13) Girl, Ivy, aged 13. Seen 28.1.41. Conjunctivitis and stye left lower eyelid. *Euphrasia* lotion, *Sulph.* 30.

Sulph. 30 repeated weekly for 3 weeks, discharged well. Seen again on 25.2.41 with a relapse. History of measles some years ago. *Euphrasia* lotion and *Morb.* 30.

Weekly doses of *Morb.* 30 were given along with *Euphrasia* locally until 1.4.41. The eyes were well within 2 weeks, but she was kept on for another 2 weeks because of her previous quick relapse. She also developed small septic pimples on her face after the first week on *Morbillinum*, an outward manifestation of elimination — the cure was going in the right direction; the more serious eye complaint was replaced by a less serious skin affliction. No return of eye trouble since.

(14) Patricia, aged 5½. Seen 27.5.41. Measles just before Christmas, bilateral conjunctivitis and cervical adenitis, and since then, pallid complexion. *Euphrasia* locally and *Morb.* 30.

10.6.41, 2 weeks later, eyes well, glands gone, looks well. *Morb.* 30. Discharged well.

(15) Minnie, 5 years old. Seen 29.5.41; bilateral blepharitis practically continuously since measles 3 years ago. Several warts below left eye and above upper lip. *Morbillinum* 30 daily for a week.

10.6.41. Blepharitis gone, warts shrinking. *Morb.* 30 daily for 3 days. First time for years that her eyes have been so well! Mother says.

(16) Girl, aged 13. Cracks both nostrils, and chronic nasal discharge for 3 months. Seen 20.8.40. The nose was treated locally with *Calendula* lotion inside, and *Calendula* ointment for the cracks outside until the end of November with no apparent improvement until *Diphtherinum* 30 was given on 19.11.40, after which it healed up within a week; another dose of *Diphtherinum* 30 was given and she was discharged, as she was of a somewhat turbulent disposition and upset everybody at the centre. Seen again on 7.1.41 with a relapse, cracked nostrils, stuffy nose, nasal discharge; nose inflamed and raw inside. History of measles in May 1940 — the first time I was told about this attack. *Morbillinum* 30 given: the nasal discharge and cracked nostrils cleared up within 7 days. *Morb.* 30 repeated. Discharged well. Seen 3 months later, the cure still held good; no further relapse yet.

This is just a small series of cases, but I only started to use *Morbillinum* early last autumn. I wish I had known about it before, when I think of the hundreds and hundreds of chronic eye inflammations I have treated during the last two decades, months and months of local treatment, relapse after relapse, the same cases invariably used to attend year in, year out, until they left school. A pitiful confession of the failure of orthodox treatment: of course conjunctivitis and blepharitis when due to dust and dirt clear up quickly enough with the local antiseptic treatment; but chronic external eye conditions remain with their victims, if they are caused by measles. Of course under-feeding, wrong feeding, has a lot to do with it and the irritation of the eye due to dust and dirt does not improve it; nor does the poor illumination in the working class homes help matters. But many of these cases had treatment for months at special eye convalescent homes, where particular attention is paid to diet: extra milk, Marmite, cod-liver oil and malt, a plentiful supply of butter, cream, eggs and oranges, extra vitamins were supplied there; in spite of this the children stayed for months — 3-6 months' stay at this home is common — while a few doses of *Morbillinum* under war conditions — a reduced fat consumption and no cod-liver oil and malt — cleared up similar chronic eye conditions in a matter of 2-3 weeks!

Now for another case. This time it was a lady in the late fifties, who has been an ardent homoeopath for years. She was evacuated officially against her wishes and while in the country came in contact with measles. She discussed the prophylaxis of measles with me and I suggested *Morbillinum* 200, 2 doses at monthly intervals. She was rather nervous at the idea of taking a measles nosode, and delayed taking it until after her next visit. When she was seen again, 4 weeks later, there was a great change in her. She had always suffered from a brilliant red nose all her life and had been very conscious of this, and had always tried to camouflage it with creams and face powders, with not too much success. The veins in her cheeks were very noticeable. When she came in through the door this time, her nose was white and of normal colour, and so were her cheeks. I laughingly asked her, had she at last found a special new varnish for covering up the colour of her nose and cheeks, when she replied with great pride that she had not used anything at all, the redness of the nose had just faded away during the last month. She had sought relief for this cosmetic trouble for years, had hoped homoeopathy would help her, but though homoeopathic medicines had helped her general health greatly, the red beacon of a nose had always stayed with her. Now it was gone. Then she told me, she had a severe attack of measles at the age of 5, and her mother had told her that she became very short-sighted after that and had to wear strong glasses for her myopia since then; her red nose had worried her ever since she began to take notice of her personal appearance in her 'teens. *Morbillinum* 200, the measles nosode, wiped this cosmetic defect out. This may not seem to be very important to most people, but it is an interesting point to remember, that enlarged veins of nose and cheeks come on after measles, and if so, that *Morbillinum* in a high potency even after half a century, will effect a cure. Still a month later the cure had held good. The nasal beacon had gone. Now one wonders whether the myopia will improve too, or has that condition become too deep-seated? It is early days to make any prophecies, but I have hopes that her sight will improve as well.

I have just seen a very sad case in a baby five months old. Her eyes were sound on 31.3.41. Then she developed measles and was 7 weeks in a fever hospital, discharged with an inflamed left eye, which on examination was congested and red all over, the left pupil was small, much smaller than the right, and also irregular and star-shaped, no alteration in shape or form when a light was directed to the pupil. It was covered with a thick turbid haze. Diagnosis: severe iritis with infection of choroid retina.

The left upper eyelid had dropped considerably and the eye was nearly closed up. A very serious condition; no wonder the eye specialist gave a very bad prognosis and foretold complete loss of sight in that eye. The mother was naturally distracted, the baby was given a dose of *Lueticum* 30, which was repeated three days later. Then I got a report from the hospital that the child had really had measles. So I changed the prescription to *Morbillinum* 100. After two doses of *Lueticum*, the upper eyelid was less prolapsed, the general redness and inflammation of the eye had gone; but the pupil was still deformed and misshapen, and there was no response to light, though there appeared to be some vision left.

The mother had been reassured; one hopes that the measles nosode will dissolve the adhesions which hold the muscles of the pupil down and that the inflammation of the retina will clear up as well. One has seen similar miracles with the correct homoeopathic medication before, and as the condition in this baby is definitely brought on by measles, the measles nosode will cure it in due course, provided the mother continues the treatment.

Homoeopathic treatment makes one more confident and sure. The law states 'like cures like', and if one finds the right remedy or series of right remedies, the cure is certain.

A few more cases of debility after measles have reported themselves lately. There is so much coming and going in the London working-class population that a continuity of observation and treatment is well-nigh impossible.

There is, for example, a mother with two boys who flits from county to county in between and pays flying visits to her husband and flat in South London. On one of these migratory attendances at her home the children were found to be suffering from some urticarial skin trouble which the Medical Officer diagnosed as an infectious kind of impetigo, for which she said hospital treatment was essential. I disagreed. The difficulty settled itself naturally by the children being sent to hospital with measles at the beginning of December, 1940. A month later the older boy, aged 2 years 8 months, weighing 29½ lb., was discharged from hospital with the identical urticaria on the lower extremities — not labelled impetigo by the hospital — and enlarged glands of the neck and slight bronchitis. Seen a month later, on February 9th, he had lost a pound in weight, had numerous enlarged and tender glands, blepharitis, sticky eyelids, and a catarrhal cough as well, generally miserable. *Morbillinum* 100 given. The mother disappeared again into the blue for five months and returned the first week of July with the child having gained 3 lb. in weight during the interval. The mother declared he had been extremely well until eight weeks ago, when he developed whooping cough which he had not been able to shake off. The sticky eyes had cleared up within a week of his last attendance at the clinic. He is being treated now with *Pertussin* for his whooping cough, which I am confident will clear it up within a few days. This child during the eight months between June 10th, 1940 and February 9th, 1941, had only gained 2 lb., even though he had been in the country during a large part of this time. But the *Morbillinum* increased his weight by 3 lb. in five months, in spite of a severe attack of whooping cough which is well noted for interfering with growth and weight.

His brother, now exactly two years old, had remained stationary in weight between August 19th, 1940 until November 21st, 1940, at 22 lb. 7 oz., even though he was in the country nearly all the time. He put on 1½ lb. in London on two doses of *Tuberculinum* 30 during the next month, when he was taken to hospital with measles. Seen two months later, he had lost 5 ounces, had blepharitis, sticky eyes in the morning and a catarrhal cough. Weight 23 lb. 9 oz. *Morbillinum* 100, one dose given.

Five months later, on his return in July, his weight was 28 lb. 14 oz., he had erupted his last four teeth without any trouble as well. The previous teeth had come through with slight catarrhal and bronchial disturbances. He is now nearly a pound overweight for his age, sturdy and firm. What a difference after the one dose of *Morbillinum*, compared to the previous 8 months. Away in the country during both these periods, food much about the same, the difference in weight came on after the dose of *Morbillinum* was given. If it was only an isolated case of improvement here and there, one would not jump to the conclusion that the correct homoeopathic medication had made such vast difference. But if you see it again and again, you cannot help but be sure of the fact that the homoeopathic remedies, if correctly applied, do alter the whole metabolism and make all the difference between a happy, jolly, healthy child and a nondescript, weakly kid who just carries on catching every disease that is going and living all the time on tonics and cod-liver oil and malt.

Thomas, aged 3 years old, weight 28 lb. 14 oz. on December 16th, 1940; going up and down in weight since July 8th, 1940, miserable with a cold and cough, enlarged tonsils. He developed measles a day or two later and came out of hospital three weeks later with a swollen face, a tongue thickly coated with white fur, very peevish and miserable. *Ant. crudum* 30, one dose, was given on these symptoms, which cleared them up rapidly. He was losing weight which he could ill afford. *Sulphur* 30 given in repeated doses, which improved his weight, so that on March 31st he weighed 31 lb., having gained 2½ lb. in two months. Three weeks later he had lost ¾ lb. again, so then, remembering the history of measles in December, he had a dose of *Morbillinum* 100; four weeks later his weight had gone up again to 31 lb. 10 oz., 1½ lb. gain during that month, which in a poor home where there are difficulties of getting suitable food for young children is quite remarkable. So the child in four months had gained 4 lb. from January 23rd, 1941, until May 26th; and his tonsils which were enormous had considerably diminished in size as well. A gain due to a few doses of *Sulphur* followed by *Morbillinum*, and the child had suffered a severe shock in the interval by being in a house which was severely damaged by a bomb. In spite of it, he had improved very much!

Baby Jean, aged 13 months, who had done well on repeated doses of *Silica*, so that she weighed 22 lb. and had 7 teeth without any disturbance, developed measles at the beginning of June, 1941. When seen again on June 19th, she was not her usual bright self, very quiet and miserable, had lost about a pound in weight. *Morbillinum* 100 given at once.

The next week she was extremely lively and happy as always, and had gained 6 oz. *Morbillinum* was repeated weekly until July 10th, when she weighed 22 lb. 3 oz., a gain of nearly 20 oz. in three weeks, plus the eruption of another tooth and four more nearly through; always cheerful and bright now.

Let me repeat once more: remember the measles serum, *Morbillinum,* in potency during the convalescence period after measles. There will be no need to send the child to the seaside or give innumerable doses of the nauseating cod-liver oil and malt mixture. This treatment is much simpler, less costly and more efficacious.

And if in an older child or even an adult you find that the individual had one or more attacks of measles, and has not been doing too well since, interpose a dose or two of *Morbillinum* 30 or higher, and then go back to the other constitutional remedies as may be necessary; and you will be surprised how quickly various states of ill-health will clear up.

CHAPTER TWENTY-FIVE

SCARLATINUM (SCARLET FEVER SERUM)

During World War I, when the women of England obeyed the call to serve their country in the hour of need by leaving their hearths and homes for the benches and the lathes, the grandparents took up their burdens again and cared for the young fledglings who might have perished otherwise. One of these grannies brought her twin grandsons to a Welfare Centre I knew — which was still somewhat of a novelty in 1916 — from three weeks of age onwards and faithfully carried out the instructions given, with great benefit to the weakly, puling infants. The old granny was of paramount interest to me because of an affliction of the eyelids which she had bravely borne without complaining for forty years or more. Her lower eyelids were completely everted, red and rheumy and inflamed like pieces of raw beef, with an excoriated and moist skin all round the eyes. She acknowledged having tried various Eye hospitals for relief of her unsightly complaint, but there was no improvement, she had given up the search for even a temporary cure of her blemish long ago. She willingly and ungrudgingly swallowed the powders and pills I gave her: *Sulphur* in various potencies, she was fat and unwieldly, slovenly and dirty. Then she had *Psorinum*, for she carried a strong odour around with her. Later we tried *Pulsatilla* and *Graphites*, but nothing was of any avail. The thing beat me completely. Granny told me it had come on after a severe attack of scarlet fever which should have been a signpost to me, but I did not have the key to the puzzle then, and the years rolled on. When the twins were seventeen years old, she loomed up once again with another child of her numerous progeny, the eyes still stark red and weeping and horrible to look at, a silent reproach to me for having failed in curing her. She bore me no ill will.

She had never expected anything else; but proudly told me of the jobs the now tall twins were holding and how well they were doing.

Nearly another decade has passed since then; another woman came along, almost the spit of the one I have described already: fat and dirty, waddling like a duck as the result of many pregnancies, lower eyelids loose and relaxed, hanging down over her cheeks like brilliant red coxcombs, extremely deaf as well, she had to be bawled at before she could understand a word. She brought an undersized lad of 10 to me with anaemia and severe conjunctivitis. I was still undaunted in spite of past failures, and on her general make-up gave her *Sulphur* 30 on March 25th, 1941. The next week the eyes were definitely improved, not so inflamed; she had not gone to the Eye hospital, as the almoner of the clinic had urged her to. Another dose of *Sulphur* 30; visited and chivied during the week by a visitor from the hospital on the report of the officious though well-meaning almoner of the clinic.

Seen again on April 22nd, eyes very much worse, had some green paint applied to her eyelids at the hospital which she disliked intensely and thereafter flatly refused to have any further local treatment. I went further into her case and discovered that the eye condition came on after a severe attack of scarlet fever when she was 37 years old, about 10 years ago. They had steadily grown worse and so had the deafness. She was 'up against it' and bore a grudge against everybody because of this blemish. Nobody could help her. It was evidently a chronic condition, the cartilage of the eyelids were much thickened and hardened. 'Since an attack of scarlet fever' now conveyed a lot to me. I was triumphant. I should be able to help her. *Scarlatinum* 200, unit dose, was given on 21st April; no local treatment advised. A week later another dose of *Scarlatinum* 200; that was on April 29th.

The mother was not seen again until June 17th, 1941, as she had slipped down some stairs during an air raid and injured her left shoulder, but the eyes were much improved and there was hardly any deafness. *Scarlatinum* 200. Three weeks later she presented herself again, almost unrecognizable, a completely changed woman, clean and spick and span in the morning, with bright cheeks not owing anything to art – clean white silk blouse, and her eyelids well – they were as normal as anybody else's. They had turned round, all the red flesh had gone, the cartilages in the eyelids were smooth and thin, and the mucous membranes barely pink, no inflammation at all! A miracle had happened in a short six weeks; she had been made new almost over night, after suffering from this disfiguring blight for over ten years. It had not prevented her from catching a second husband though in the interval!

Motherlike, she had nothing to say about her own cure; she was the fierce lioness guarding her own cub who was to be snatched away from her arms by the relentless act of an impersonal civic authority, 'forcibly evacuated as living in unsuitable surroundings in a danger area', was the official language, 'and suffering in health in consequence'. Neither mother nor boy saw it that way; they loved one another and preferred to live and, if necessary, to die together.

Whether she will prevail against authority is doubtful; but the return to normal of her eyes and the loss of an unsightly blemish was completely swamped for her by the threatened loss of her own child.

The power of the infinitesimal over a definite physical lesion in a very short time, leaves one almost breathless. In looking up the orthodox textbooks on treatment of Ectropion, or eversion of the eyelids, as this complaint is called, one finds that not much hope is given of curing it. Local treatment by means of caustics such as silver nitrate, etc., is advised, and if that does not help, a choice of operations is given as the only ultimate cure; even that is faintly decried. One has seen a number of these unsightly inflamed everted eyelids, usually in people of the lower order, tramps and folks who reside in unsavoury lodging-houses, evidently people who do not get enough suitable food of the right kind. A deficiency disease perhaps in some instances. And yet how quickly curable, if you know how, if you have the key to unlock the door to the temple of health.

Scarlet fever serum inoculation has been tried recently as a prophylactic, a prevention against scarlet fever, with not always too great a success, judging from some instances I have come across.

Two young lads under ten, sons of a well-known consultant physician, were pupils in a famous expensive boarding school; scarlet fever broke out and the whole school was inoculated against scarlet fever; none of the parents were asked for permission, of course, that goes without saying. Medical tyranny and Hitlerism will have to be fought here in England as well as on the Continent. The result of this inoculation of this doctor's two sons, was unforseen and somewhat tragic as regards the progress of their schooling and their studies. They both developed high temperatures and a most irritating and disconcerting urticarial eruption all over the arms and the body which kept them awake and scratching day and night. Calamine lotion had to be applied by the pint, and it did not ease a scrap, the temperature kept up for weeks. The lads got thinner and thinner, in spite of best expert advice; they were brought home to their parents and for 16 weeks they were in bed suffering untold agonies. Their mother, who told me, took it all as a matter of course, and she prided herself on being a practical and intelligent woman!

The scarlet fever serum is a powerful agent in producing a long lasting urticaria, therefore it should be remembered as a standby in urticiaria which will not yield to other means, provided it is given in a high dilution.

It should and will also act curatively in ailments left after scarlet fever. Kidney diseases, albuminuria, ear diseases following on scarlet fever, and so on, such as the case I described just now, whose deafness of middle-ear origin following on the infection of the eustachian canal from scarlet fever was completely cured by a few doses of *Scarlatinum*, as well as the condition of the eyelids.

Dr. J. H. Clarke recommends *Scarlatinum* or scarlet-fever-serum nosode, in a high dilution as a preventive of scarlet fever. I have never had occasion to try it. I have always followed Hahnemann's suggestion, who advised *Belladonna* as the best prophylactic against scarlet fever, which I have proved to be correct over and over again.

A young girl of 16 developed scarlet fever in a mild form some twenty years ago. I gave her *Bell.* 200 two hourly; the rash and throat disappeared in 48 hours, and she was well in a few days. Several younger brothers and sisters in the house who were contacts were all given *Bell.* 30 three times daily and none of the other contacts developed scarlet fever.

Several times during a period of six years or more I was providential in preventing the spread of scarlet fever in a couple of day nurseries which were under my care. *Bell.* 30, night and morning was given as a routine for a week, as soon as a case of scarlet fever was reported as having occurred in the families of any of the children. Result, no scarlet fever developed. And no violent reactions occurred either as the result of taking *Belladonna*.

Is this not a much wiser and more commonsense proceeding than overdosing and crippling the unfortunate children for weeks after huge doses of scarlet fever serum?

I just recall another case of discharging ear in a young child following scarlet fever. She had been 13 weeks or more in a fever hospital with it and her ear was very offensive and running freely. *Scarlatinum* 200 cleared it up in a fortnight and I have known these cases of ear discharge, dating back to scarlet fever, go on for months and months, and even years.

Another girl of 10 who was suffering from bed-wetting and had a foul smelling discharge from her ears due to scarlet fever, was given weekly doses of *Scarlatinum* 200 and the ear cleared up effectively in a month. It had gone on for a year previously, and the bed-wetting disappeared as well in three or four weeks, though she had suffered from it for more than five years.

A girl of 14 some years ago came up with static albuminuria, after scarlet fever. Albuminuria which came on as soon as she got up from her bed in the morning and stayed with her as long as she was up and about; her legs were swollen to her knees. *Scarlatinum* 200 in weekly doses soon put her right.

These are just some of the cases I can recall, and when I compare the results I have had with this remedy whenever it was indicated, with those I had when I prescribed the orthodox treatment, such as acid tonics or iron mixtures or cod liver oil and malt, with convalescence at the seaside, well — there is no comparison really. With this remedy, *Scarlatinum* in a high potency, you just cured these cases, rapidly, quickly, imperceptibly, almost overnight — and with the orthodox way of 'cure' — well, it was just a parody of the word. They went on feeling seedy and never quite the thing, there was never 'this joy of living' and of being on top of the world, such as a healthy individual should experience.

Nosodes or remedies made from the serum of a particular disease, are wonderful remedial agents and should not be neglected by homoeopaths.

CHAPTER TWENTY-SIX

MENTAL DISEASE AND HOMOEOPATHY

A friend of mine was idly going through one of my Materia Medica books, when she suddenly exclaimed: 'What peculiar symptoms one finds in your remedies. Can you really cure people with these ideas?' I glanced over her shoulder to see what remedy she had been reading and found that it was *Thuja*. 'This is not so difficult to answer,' I replied; 'thereby hangs a tale' — and here it is.

Several times in my life it has been my fate to live in close contact with mentally weak or diseased people for months on end. And very attractive people they proved to be. They were like children, not hiding their innermost thoughts, but frank — often brutally so — in their likes and dislikes and refreshingly simple. Humour them, encourage them, draw them out and they were easily guided and drawn away from their pet evil and depressing thoughts. I used to collect and write down some of their peculiarities, their funny ideas and delusions. I was not allowed to treat them homoeopathically, though I was itching to do so. I used to pore over my books, my Repertory and my Materia Medica and write in the margins 'Mr. A' or 'Mr. B', to remind me of the person who showed these outlandish, often laughable, symptoms.

There was a young man, the only son of his parents, alas! He could never pass a horse in the street; he would kneel down in the street behind the horse's tail and pray. He had religious mania, why he should kneel down by a horse, I do not know; it was very disconcerting, anyway, to go out with him. In those days the horse was a common object in the streets of London, not a rarity. So he had to be shut up, and he used to be found always in corners kneeling down and praying. Once he managed to escape and climbed over the high wall of the institution, in order to make for home. But he did not get far, the first horse he met distracted his attention, and he was caught again quite quickly, kneeling at the tail of a horse, praying. Kent's Repertory gives several remedies under the symptom, 'Kneeling and praying'; *Ars., Nat. sulph. Stramonium* and *Veratrum.* Curiously enough there is a rubric even: 'insists upon saying his prayers at the tail of his horse — *Euphorbium.*'

Stramonium and *Veratrum* are remedies which with *Hyoscyamus* would empty our asylums of more than 75 per cent of their inmates in a short time; and it is a crying shame that there are no homoeopathic institutions in this country. In the United States, I believe, there are large asylums, where the patients are treated homoeopathically, and where the recovery rate is much higher than in the orthodox institutions.

I wish I could tell you that I had cured this young man of his religious mania, but I was unable to give him anything but allopathic remedies, and when I left after six months, he was still there. Nowadays, of course, if I had the chance again, I should slip *Stramonium* or *Veratrum*, or whichever remedy was indicated, into his tea, and chance being discovered. I only studied and classified temperaments and peculiarities then.

There was another middle-aged man in that hospital. His father was a well-known professor. I do not remember how his son went off the rails, he appeared quite sane, until you mentioned 'policemen'; then he always got violent — he thought he *saw policemen* coming into the house, if he was at home with his parents. The remedies for this delusion would have been, if I had had the chance to treat him, again *Hyoscyamus* or *Kali bromide*, of course in potency. Curiously enough they often gave *Hyoscyamus* in material doses in this hospital — that is, they used the concentrated alkaloid Hyoscine hydrobrom, in $\frac{1}{100}$ grain doses. It was given as a sleeping draught in beer to the men and in tea to the women — unbeknown to them. It made them sleep and quietened them, it is true, but it was given for its physiological actions. It would have worked much better and gone much deeper and really cured — that is, removed the delusions and restored the patients' mentality — if it had been given in minute doses, when it would act on a higher plane than the physical.

Unfortunately it is difficult, almost impossible, to treat mental patients in their homes. They want careful handling, friendly and kindly supervision, by people who understand mental kinks. This means a specially trained staff who are firm with them when they get excited, yet not brutal. Fresh air, sleeping out-of-doors, rambling in gardens and woods of institutions, out-of-door occupations, all this is necessary. It takes time to cure a diseased mind, often weeks and months, and, during this process of slow recovery, patients may slide back and may commit acts dangerous to themselves and others, and therefore supervision under kindly control is necessary. Alas, as I said before, that Homoeopathy is not given a chance to hold out a helping hand to these poor bewildered souls.

But I am a long time coming to my tale. The symptom my friend found so impossible and ludicrous was docketed under: '*Thinks she is made of glass*' and marked: *Thuja*. My thoughts flew back to this very asylum I have been talking of just now, and I recalled the quaint figure of a middle-aged man, who was never known to speak to anybody; he was always standing about as if he was watching for something, or somebody, and if anybody came near him, he quickly drew out of their way, so that nobody should touch him. He had been an inmate for years. The one outstanding peculiarity about him was, he was enormously fat. I asked the medical superintendent about this patient, and he laughingly replied: 'Just feel him the next time you go round.' I made it my business to do so and to my surprise found he was padded with layers and layers of newspapers and journals. No newspaper was safe from him, we never saw any newspapers in the male wing, he always pounced on any paper he found lying about, and added it to his store round his body. It was not that he was cold; no, he thought he was so brittle that he would break unless he protected himself with papers. He was made of glass and must therefore not be touched, unless he had these layers of papers round him, which made him feel safe! You see, this symptom was not so out-of-the-way after all. I have come across it clinically in a patient, a well authenticated case. The whole staff of the asylum knew about this man's peculiarity, and his whims. Nothing was done for him, except he might indulge himself in winding papers round himself. Oh! I wished so much I could have given him *Thuja*, so as to prove to myself that it was possible to cure mentally afflicted persons.

I have met these symptoms since, in not such a pronounced form, in a young girl, barely three years old, and I was able to eradicate it completely. This little girl from South London was a 'bad doer' weighed about 21 lb. at three years of age, had no appetite, had been given all kinds of tonics, without any result. She had this great peculiarity: she hated anybody to touch her; even her mother dare not touch her. She would not allow herself to be picked up, and there were frightful scenes when she had to be dressed and undressed night and morning. She would not sit on her mother's lap even, she played about quite happily, by herself, if she was left alone. The mother told me little Ann had said to her that she would break if anybody touched her. I gave her *Thuja* in repeated doses, first in the 6th potency and later in the thirtieth, and she put on weight very rapidly, her appetite improved, and she even allowed herself to be dressed without tears. She always remained a self-possessed madam, as long as I knew her, which was for about a year — always like the cat that walked by herself; but she forgot in the end that she would break in two if she were touched. Another of my little 'difficult children' put right by Homoeopathy.

I am sure if that gentleman in the asylum had been given *Thuja* he would have lost this strange idea of 'being made of glass', and, who knows, he might have been able to return to the bosom of his family — a mentally sound man, for barring this one delusion which obtruded upon everything in his life, there was nothing else wrong. Remove this '*idée fixe*' and there would have been once more a sound mind in a sound body. Do not say, I am making a statement without a solid backing of truth. Our Law says: 'like cures like'. On the one hand you have this symptom, which was found in a healthy 'prover' and on the other side you have the identical symptoms in the sick person; and from past innumerable clinical experiences of mine as well as those of all the other homoeopathic doctors, past and present, I know this delusion will disappear, if *Thuja* is given. This is 'positive therapy', and a certain school in France would like to change the name 'Homoeopathy' to 'Positive Therapeutics'; and they are not far wrong. For 'we know' and we can foretell, what is going to happen, if the right remedy is given, and we know in many cases which is the right curative remedy and the reason why.

Have I ever cured a mental patient? I certainly have, and in an astonishingly short period, too. Let me tell you about it.

An elderly woman came into the surgery carrying a three weeks old baby, behind her trailed the mother of the baby, looking lost and bewildered. She, that is the young mother, sat down in a corner and took no further notice of the proceedings. The grandmother complained, she had been like this ever since the confinement; she would not look after the baby, or the husband, or the flat. She just sat and moped, as I saw her, did not answer when spoken to, did not stir. She might lift her head and look at the person who addressed her, with a suspicious, startled look, that was all the sign she gave of having understood what was being said to her. Her husband had tried everything, coaxing and endearments, he had even beaten her; it was not the slightest use. She would not work or do anything at all. She was just like a dummy figure. The grandmother had to look after the baby, or it would have starved. What she was to do, she did not know. I told her to return the next day and I should try and help her. The next day, no Mrs. B. came. I was sure she had been removed to the local Infirmary for observation, before being certified insane. I had diagnosed her as a case of puerperal insanity, due to shock at the birth — a fairly common incident — and it takes quite six to nine months before these unfortunate women recover, as a rule, under ordinary treatment. I was sorry, of course, for I hoped that I could have done something for her. A week later there was the same procession again, granny with the baby, and the miserable, dreamy mentally afflicted mother. Granny informed me she had taken her to the family doctor who advised removal to the asylum, as nothing else would do any good; she would have to be certified. Granny was somewhat reluctant to do this and then remembering my offer, had come back to me for further advice. I gave the patient some *Sulphur* 10*m*, and as she was very poor, told the old lady to carry on as before; of course, if the young woman got worse, she was to send her to the institution. I was somewhat anxious naturally, these patients sometimes commit murder and kill the unconscious cause of their trouble, the baby. The following week the procession came in again, this time with this difference: that the young woman carried the baby and grandma walked behind. The mother timidly, blushing slightly, offered the baby for examination and granny explained that she had suddenly started the day after the previous visit to take an interest in the baby and asked to be allowed to look after it herself. Granny was still somewhat anxious, but very pleased at this unexpected change. The week after, there was no granny, mother and baby came in by themselves. She looked after baby and the house and the husband, all by herself, somewhat awkwardly and somewhat slowly still, but she managed it all without help from anybody. And from henceforth, there was no looking back, but a steady improvement. She lost her pallid, anaemic look, the colour came back, she took an interest and a great interest too, in herself, her personal appearance, and her baby. There could not have been a prouder and happier mother! A case of puerperal insanity cured within a day or two — the change began within twenty-four hours — instead of six to nine months, as the textbooks tell you, and the medical officers in mental institutions will tell you, and they have them under their care, so they should know.

And this woman never looked back, and it was not just a

flash in the pan, but a genuine recovery. I saw her and the child for close on two years, and watched for any signs of recurrence with impartial interest. True, it was an early case of puerperal insanity, seen in the early days; but they are usually admitted to the hospitals very soon after the confinement as nothing but institutional care is any good. Why, I ask again, not give Homoeopathy a chance and put aside a few cases of acute insanity, such as this, and experiment with homoeopathic remedies? The doses are so small, they could not do any harm, and if given with insight and knowledge, would cure many a case which now lingers inside the walls of a mental institution.

CHAPTER TWENTY-SEVEN

NERVOUS DISORDERS

A vivid description of acute insanity is given in the Book of Books, which I will quote:—

'The king spake, and said, Is not this great Babylon, that I have built for the house of the kingdom by the might of my power, and for the honour of my majesty?

'While the word was in the King's mouth, there fell a voice from heaven, saying, O king Nebuchadnezzar, to thee it is spoken; The kingdom is departed from thee.

'And they shall drive thee from men, and thy dwelling shall be with the beasts of the field: they shall make thee to eat grass as oxen, and seven times shall pass over thee, until thou know that the most High ruleth in the kingdom of men, and giveth it to whomsoever he will.

'The same hour was the thing fulfilled upon Nebuchadnezzar: and he was driven from men, and did eat grass as oxen, and his body was wet with the dew of heaven, till his hairs were grown like eagles' feathers, and his nails like birds' claws.

'And at the end of the days I Nebuchadnezzar lifted up mine eyes unto heaven, and mine understanding returned unto me, and I blessed the most High ... At the same time my reason returned to me ... and my counsellors and my lords sought unto me; and I was established in my kingdom ... Now I Nebuchadnezzar praise and extol and honour the King of heaven ... and those that walk in pride he is able to abase.'

This ancient king suffered from Megalomania or a swollen head and this led to his undoing, his mind became clouded, and he behaved like an animal, lived with them in the open-air, ate like them for seven years, until he recognized the power of a higher being, and in all humility confessed his sin of spiritual pride; then he became rational once more.

There are many causes for this break-down in mental reasoning power. Fear and worry and anxiety are a common cause of acute mental trouble and mental diseases could be cured many times, if taken in time in the early stages before the mind has become too clouded to respond to appropriate treatment, at a place, where they understand how to deal with them; for the majority of folks are afraid of diseased minds and run miles rather than face them.

I came across such a case the other day; this was an acute break-down, and the local practitioner, called in by the frightened mother, gave a very bad diagnosis, told her that her daughter, aged under thirty, was finished, that it was quite hopeless, her brain had gone completely. Naturally the mother believed him; fortunately for her and the poor afflicted daughter, the local G.P. would not certify her or send her into the Municipal hospital for observation. He passed on the responsibility to me.

The history was an alarming one, I must admit. She had been suffering from nocturnal epileptic fits for several years, which were not controlled by Luminal, she had these night fits at least three or four times a week, sometimes oftener, until the previous week, when these fits were almost continuous, going from one fit into another all night long. During the day she was vacant, refused to answer, would not speak at all, refused to touch food, vomited if any food was pressed on her, and she was incontinent as well. This went from bad to worse for several days. She lived miles away from anywhere, in the depths of the country; so she was brought up to town in an ambulance and taken to a Home where they take borderline cases at a reasonable fee. A great consideration this!

She was given small doses of *Hyoscyamus* which is one of the remedies for nocturnal epilepsy, and when I saw her she was quiet and had had no fits since the *Hyoscyamus* had been given. She was sullen, suspicious, only answered 'yes', when spoken to, which was somewhat of an improvement as compared with the state she had been in for three days before. The *Hyoscyamus* had done this at once. She was left to the kind care of competent nurses in a ground-floor room, where she could do herself no damage. The report for the first thirty-six hours was a somewhat serious one; she became extremely violent during the first night and shouted and struggled so that six people were required to hold her down; and *Hyoscyamus* $\frac{1}{100}$ gr. or 2x given hypodermically was necessary to quieten her. There was a similar scene the next night, and again *Hyoscyamus* 2x was given with a quietening effect. The second morning she was still irrational, shouted at intervals 'I want to − I want to', without saying what she wanted. Then she would flop on the floor and crawl on all fours round and round the room. All the furniture was removed, and she was allowed to amuse herself crawling to and fro, while *Hyoscyamus* 30 was given 4 hourly.

The third day she woke up and asked with a puzzled expression: 'How old am I?' and when told she was nearly 30, she did not begin her crawling again, but stayed quietly in bed and there were no further scenes, no violent rages, no exhausting struggles. She took her food, whatever was given to her, and she behaved like a tired but otherwise rational being, sleeping a great deal both by day and night. She must have been exhausted after the continuous fits and her violence for the past week. Then her period came on, and this explained the violence of the attack; for the days before the monthly period often produce a violent explosion in mental cases. Everything settled down then; she ate well, she enjoyed her food; all the bodily functions worked well and normally and she answered rationally, she took an interest in her surroundings; there were no further fits, no further attacks of violence. What more could you expect?

The acute attack, once proper care and attention were given and once the right remedy was found, passed in a few short days. After the first dose of *Hyoscyamus* 30 the fits ceased and the incontinence stopped. These had lasted, as I said, for six days; but the hang-over after the epileptic explosion lasted for forty-eight hours, and was controlled by two doses of *Hyoscyamus* in a low potency and further doses of *Hyoscyamus* high.

The nurses of the Home were astonished how rapidly the attack passed and how quickly she became rational. She will have to stay in the Home for several weeks and will have to be watched and kept quiet, live an orderly, well regulated life on a proper non-meat diet, and on homoeopathic medication and with interesting manual occupation in the kitchen and in the garden one can guarantee that there will be no further acute attacks of brainstorms. The epileptic attacks, if and when the right remedy for this constitutional complaint is found, will eventually be controlled; but this may mean months of treatment. Homoeopathy takes a long time to build up a person's constitution, it does not do to lose patience. The first doctor's pessimistic verdict has been proved wrong, thanks to Homoeopathy, but what a lot of harm could have been done, if the mother had taken his word for gospel and the poor child had gone to a mental ward for observation. Another great essential is to find a Home where the instructions of a homoeopathic physician are correctly carried out, and where no sleeping draughts and no drugs are given which destroy the brain cells and the reasoning power of the poor mental wreck.

King Nebuchadnezzar in the Bible story only got his reason back because he followed his inclination, lived in the open-air on a non-meat diet, and was not given any drugs. I guarantee if he had been kept in a modern institution behind lock and key, continually hearing the rattle of keys and kept under drugs, he would never have got back his reason. Modern treatment seems very odd to me. A sane child is not disciplined, must not be repressed under any condition, must be allowed to follow his own inclination, and when he grows up and when he becomes mentally deranged from too much licence being given to him, preventive treatment is then applied to him, he is repressed by large doses of drugs and kept forever — nearly always it means life-long imprisonment — in a mental hospital. Why not teach discipline in the early days of childhood and point out the importance of the repression of anti-social qualities?

Let me add some further remarks about the patient I have been talking about. She had been suffering for four years from attacks of so-called night epilepsy and had been examined by many different doctors in Ireland and London. Some suggested pressure on the brain, others suggested brain tumour, she had all kinds of tests performed on her which showed no evidence of any disease.

During the whole of the time she had been heavily dosed with increasing doses of the most commonly used of the Barbiturate series.

This drug never controlled the fits; it only made her heavy and stupid, forgetful and sleepless. She was given *Thuja* 200 when first seen, then later *Lyc.* 6 t.d.s., taken off all flesh diet and put on a vegetarian diet and did extremely well. Played golf, slept well at night and without any sign of a fit. Then after over two months of peace and steady progress, suddenly there was this violent outbreak which I described at the beginning.

The doctor in the country gave her an injection while she was so violent; she was found to be bruised all over, when she returned to her senses.

For three whole months now there has been no return of any trouble; no fits, no fear of a fit even. She has gone back to her normal occupation, long ago, and is working harder than she has for months and is putting her whole heart and soul into it.

She is living on a purely vegetarian diet, sleeping exceedingly well without any extraneous aid, and as her mother wrote: 'She is years younger, marvellously improved, you would not know her as the same girl. What a wonderful thing homoeopathy is.'

Yes, even in Mental diseases homoeopathy helps; and it need not take seven years either as was the case with King Nebuchadnezzar.

Report received recently, 'that this young girl has remained well during the last four years.'

NERVE TROUBLE

What makes people go to the doctor? Usually it is pain and they want something to remove it. Unfortunately in the last few years the curse of self drugging has spread amongst rich and poor, so much so that pain by itself does not often bring a sufferer to the physician, as everybody takes some popular brand or another of an aceto-salicylic acid preparation for the alleviation of suffering. And thus the cause of the pain is not discovered, the pain is only suppressed, and the actual disease which produced the pain originally goes on unchecked, and when the patient comes to the doctor at last after years of self-drugging, following the advice of the widely advertised drug preparations which confront you from every hoarding, 'Take so and so for your headache', such and such a drug 'for insomnia or any other pain you may complain of' — then the disease is often so far advanced that very little can be done.

The other thing which brings a patient to his doctor, he feels run down and wants a tonic, a bottle of medicine — the cult of the tonic is difficult to kill; very often all that is needed is more rest, more fresh air, simpler food of the right kind, properly cooked and less in quantity.

But besides these folk, who are continually drugging themselves with pain-killing dopes and tonic mixtures from the doctors' medicine shelves, or more frequently still from the shelves of the dispensing chemists, there are a certain minority who look ill and are evidently in need of treatment and yet stoutly maintain there is nothing wrong with them. What are you to do with that class? The best way to find out what to do for people is to watch and observe them carefully; the majority are dumb, they do not know what ails them or how to explain themselves, and the best method is to see people under all sorts of conditions, live with them in fact, and then you can frequently make quite brilliant cures in apparently obscure cases — in cases where the person concerned did not know even, he or she was ill.

Many people are psychological misfits, they are ill, their minds are wrong, their nerves are out of order and they do not know it. I came across such a case in my own immediate surroundings. A new domestic came to me highly recommended by friends; I was warned that she had to be gently handled, she took fright easily, did not like to be scolded, that she would not complain, but would rather cut and run if things did not please her. Good servants are like precious gold these days, they have to be searched for, and if found, have to be cossetted and studied. This woman was middle-aged, looked very white and anaemic and thin; but she declared she had always been that colour, never been any different, and that she felt perfectly well.

Our house is always extremely well aired and rather on the cool side, all the windows are kept open; so very shortly the treasure developed a cold. She was sneezing, snivelling, coughing, had a slightly flushed face; so she was sent home to bed and given some *Pulsatilla* 6 t.d.s. This cleared up the fever and chills rapidly in a couple of days; but she continued to look white and tired and complained of having a lot to do. I watched her for some weeks for further indications; and gradually I discovered the following characteristics. She was muddle-headed, confused and unable to concentrate. She was always in a hurry and yet could never get finished. Late in the evening she was still cleaning and scouring though she had been at it all day. On coming into the house one found a tin of metal polish in one room, some furniture polish in another; a duster on the stairs, soap in one corner, the broom in another, dirty crockery was left everywhere until late in the evening. One week the silver would not be polished, another week the kitchen was left dirty, always something forgotten, and yet she was always rushing about as if her very life depended on it. She started the bits of personal linen she had to wash out on a Monday morning, by the Saturday they were still lying about rough dried and unironed. A thoroughly aggravating person. An evil star made us have a small dinner party. She was all hurry and flurry and scurry dashing here, there and everywhere picking up one thing, putting it down, washing two potatoes, then doing a few vegetables, then going back to the potatoes, then starting the meat, and so on. The result was, of course, disastrous, tepid soup, half boiled potatoes, nasty tepid vegetables, over cooked meat, half cold coffee, and yet the dinner was an hour late. She was like a cricket, hopping about, chirping and chirping, frightfully busy, full of many words and nothing to show for it. What could be done about it? Was I to send her to a psycho-analyst, for him to discover the reasons for this confusion of mind? And how would he set about to cure it? This was a psychological fault, obviously; the woman was able to work and most willing to oblige and spent hours pottering about. For example she spent nearly three hours sweeping a few inches of snow from the front door steps down the garden path!

I do not know what the psychologist would have advised, and how to bridge over this discontinuity of mind, the willingness to work and the confusion and the bother over it! She was only a working woman, and there was no money in it, and psycho-analysis takes much time and much money; and here there was neither time nor money. So we tried what homoeopathy could do; I did some hunting around, looking up and comparing remedies in various materia medica books; and eventually I found it all under an almost unknown remedy. *Centaurea tagana*, one of the centauries, which are closely allied to the thistles, this *Centaurea* produced the same stupidity and confusion of mind in one of the provers; this loss of commonsense, this slowness over trifling jobs, this tiredness after doing practically nothing; leaving things unfinished and starting something else before the first job was done.

I think on looking round, many more people require a few doses of *Centaurea* than you think. What about the British workman and the British painter? Woe unto you if you have a few of this tribe in your house. They pull the whole house upside down, leave everything unfinished for days and weeks; floors up everywhere, walls half stripped, ceilings half done, etc., etc!

The *Centaurea tagana* was given in the unit dose and in the 30th potency. The pretext was that she had a slight irritating, tickling, nervous cough which required attention. I dared not tell her of course that her manner of doing her work required changing. We watched, after the dose had been given, with some misgivings, I must own. You cannot alter the ways of a person, surely, I was told. Slowly, but quite unmistakably the change took place; she became quicker in her movements, she got more done in a shorter time; there was not the same desperate rushing about; the movements became quieter, she accomplished more; she was less fractious, less tired, less timid, did not look so frightened. The change was even remarked upon by visitors to the house. 'You have a new maid since my last visit a month ago.' And they would hardly believe it was the same girl; she has such a good colour, such a good complexion and she used to be so pale and look so distrait and so worried. And now she is so calm and serene. The *Centaurea* was repeated at monthly intervals with great success, then the war came along and she fled from London with the rest; but in 1946 she returned, reporting how well she felt and asking to be taken back.

Yes, the whole make-up of a person can be altered by the correctly applied remedy — Homoeopathy can beat psychology. There are many difficulties in the way, first there is the patient. How many people *know themselves*? There was a saying of a Greek philosopher to his disciples: 'Man know Thyself,' and after this self-knowledge has been acquired, set to and live up to it, alter yourself, train yourself and grow in wisdom and stature. If a person does not know herself, has never found out what the secret mainsprings of her life are, what makes her like and dislike certain things and people; why she does certain things in a certain way, can she expect to be changed, to be made whole? The psychologist is on the right track; he teaches people to think, to track down the mental cause of a trouble, of an affliction. But does he go far enough? Has he got anything else to offer, except words and explanations? I consider the homoeopath goes deeper, he digs out the cause of the trouble in the sick individual, or tries to, if the patient will let him help. And then the homoeopath has hundreds of remedies in mild doses to choose from, which have been tried out first on healthy individuals, and certain definite reactions have been produced, in people while they were in a state of health; and the homoeopathic physician knows that the sick organism which presents a certain range of symptoms can be cured by the similar remedy or remedies in succession. He is so sure of his ground, and if he sees a certain combination of symptoms and recognizes them, he knows and he can predict that the patient will be cured. It may take time, granted:— specially in people who have been ill for years and do not know what it is to feel well and strong. And then the other difficulty is, after assembling all the symptoms from the sick individual, if he is willing to co-operate, is one able to find the *'summum bonum'*, the desired goal, the single drug, which fits the patient in question. It depends on the knowledge of the physician, there are hundreds to choose from. Some may be like, some more similar, it is almost impossible to find the most similar, the most like remedy. Frequently the doctor has to be satisfied with the second best, a *somewhat* similar remedy, or even a combination of closely related and similar remedies and some of our healers and doctors, both in England and on the Continent, make excellent cures with alternating drugs. People do present such problems these days, they have had so many different inoculations, vaccinations and serums; such a mixture of chronic diseases handed down to them through their ancestors, and on top of this most have a variety of badly treated acute infectious diseases on their score sheets, which have to be taken into account. Therefore one has to consider all the past chronic infections in each case.

But the homoeopath is better equipped than the rest of orthodox and unorthodox practitioners. He has a law of cure, that like cures like, remedies which have been tried out by the acid tests of experiment on the healthy prover, not in the laboratory, not in test-tubes, but on a living, breathing, thinking, healthy person. And if he finds the right remedy, the change is evident to everybody, there is no doubt about it. It is better than bottles of tonic, better than many tons of pain-killing dope, injections or inoculations.

I saw another case of psychological trouble; a case of

nerves. She was a woman in the middle forties, a nurse who had nursed and helped to cure a chronic case of mine some twenty odd years ago. She had been abroad in the interval and after many vicissitudes had drifted back to London. In 1929 she had an ovarian cyst and the appendix removed; ever since had never got rid of a pain on the left side of the abdomen. This pain was the typical 'Mittelschmerz' of the German gynaecologist. It came on right in the middle between the periods, not during or before or after periods; but for a definite time between the periods, about six to eight days after the periods and lasted until eight days before the next period. It was said to be nerves; it was always better on holidays and when she was resting. Unfortunately it was necessary for her to earn her living as a nurse and she had to lift and carry patients, which did not improve matters. The only advice she had been given was to grin and bear the pain or go back to the surgeon for him to find out what the pain was due to. It might be adhesions after the previous operation! This did not appeal to her as the last operation had cost her a great deal of money, she had been unable to work for nearly a year; and as she was in a comfortable job at the moment, she did not wish to give it up. And yet there was this constantly recurring pain, which undermined her health and her nerves. She looked dragged and old, very thin and emaciated and had an unhealthy greyish colour. I hardly recognized her after twenty years, she used to be a bonny, lively happy-go-lucky Irish colleen, and now this miserable middle-aged woman. She got so tired when walking; and there was also pressure on the bladder, she had frequency of micturition with the pains, so that she was afraid to venture far.

The pain was worse during micturition, across abdomen from hip to hip, and was worse also when the urge to pass water came on; she had been vaccinated twice; and there was the history of an ovarian cyst. Three definite symptoms pointing to *Thuja*; and *Thuja* 30 was prescribed.

Seen a month later, the period was a fortnight late, she was sleeping better and feeling better, much less tired and looked less dragged already. She had been for a long walk the previous day and had no pains in the abdomen. Repeat *Thuja* 30 to be followed by *Pulsatilla* 12 three times a day.

Seen three weeks later, had overlifted herself by trying to balance by herself a very heavy patient. Pain and tenderness in sacrum. I manipulated the back and advised exercises for strengthening gluteal and sacral muscles — there was no frequency of micturition now, the uterus *which was retroverted at the first visit, had corrected itself.*

Arnica 30 prescribed for the effects of the strain and the overlifting. Seen two weeks later, back was quite recovered; to continue *Pulsatilla* 12 three times a day. *Pulsatilla* was given, as she liked sympathy, could not eat fat, got easily depressed and wept quietly, the tears were very near the surface; pain in the abdomen gone in less than two months and she had had this pain for nine years, ever since her operation!!

Seen again four weeks later; feels different altogether, has been going out to dances over the Christmas and enjoyed herself, which she had not been able to do for ten years! She is still very thin and lanky, 5 ft. 10 in. in height and only weighs 9 st. 4 lb. To put on more weight, drink one pint of milk daily, eat two or three eggs, she cannot take cream; but she is to take bran for tendency to constipation and for piles. *Hamamelis* ointment for piles.

I did not see her for nearly two months, she felt so much better; she feels so well, as if walking on air, goes out on every possible occasion, goes to parties and dances. No frequency of micturition, no back-ache, no pain in the abdomen. The Mittelschmerz is a thing of the past. She used to suffer from terrible depression, this was the first time she mentioned this, she felt like murdering people, she felt so ill, that she could almost do away with herself as she saw no way out of it; the constant drag, the constant pain; no doctor could help her before. She was told to go to the psychologist, as she was suffering from nerves and repression of sex, etc. —

Her face is not nearly so livid, her eyes look bright and clear, *Sulphur* 30 given for haemorrhoids, as these irritate during the period.

A week later she rang up in great consternation, as the pain in the ovary and the discomfort had returned, also the pain in the bladder and the frequency, she is also more tired. She got a shock when all these old symptoms from which she had been free for nearly five months returned again. I reassured her, said it was due to the stirring up from *Sulphur* 30 and antidoted it by returning again to *Pulsatilla* 12 which evidently was still her remedy.

Since then I have learned that she is extremely well, she has no further symptoms, no further pain, no more discomfort, she is putting on weight. She also went to her ophthalmic surgeon who was extremely astonished to find that her eyesight had improved so much, she could read better and her vision was back again to what it was some four or five years ago. 50 per cent improvement, he said.

This woman was suffering from nerves due to retroversion of the uterus and a chronic internal pain which preyed on her mind and for which no other treatment was suggested except a problematic operation. Nine years of suffering. Nine years of mind pain, of psychological anxiety, fear of losing her job owing to ill-health. A case of nerves. She had not been near a doctor for herself for years as nobody had suggested anything constructive until she remembered homoeopathy. And then a rapid cure. She came prepared to be helped, prepared to be honest and open about her ailments and symptoms.

The result was peace and comfort, another patient saved from the operating table, saved from a futile operation, and the case of nerves was cured, not by suggestion, not by faith; but by the indicated remedies. The pain went, the retroverted uterus righted itself and the vision improved; and the homoeopathic remedy built up the health and strength of one of the world's workers, who depended on her own efforts to keep going. Find out the psychologic make-up of a person, or as Hahnemann puts it, get the mental symptoms clearly differentiated and you will get a cure.

CHAPTER TWENTY-EIGHT

WHAT IS CURABLE IN MEDICINE

What is curable in medicine varies in each age, each generation, indeed almost in each decade. The tide of curability ebbs and flows according to the opinions held at the time by the then exponents of the Art of Medicine. Sometimes the ability of curing recedes far out into the ocean of vague theories, leaving the doctors floundering amidst the sandbanks of their own lack of understanding; then in the fulness of time, the tide of knowledge comes rushing back with great force, overwhelming the men looking for hidden treasures in the treacherous sands instead of looking up and ahead.

I consider medical training and education lacks continuity of thought and is apt to leave men and women stranded on little islets of ideas planted in their minds by their respective teachers.

How different is the legal mind, the legal training: 'This, I perceive,' said Cicero in *De Legibus*, lib. II, c. 4 — 'was the opinion of the wisest man that law was not invented by the human mind, nor is a decree of the people; but is something eternal which guides the whole world, the wisdom commanding and forbidding. Hence they said that the principal and ultimate law was the mind of God, through reason, enjoying or forbidding everything.'

The legal training depends on continuity of thought, goes back along the centuries and each legal case and decision is noted and studied and referred to again and again; old legal books are valuable as books of reference; in chambers and in court, the judges, counsels and solicitors consult past statutes, decrees and judgments. A lawyer may be long-winded, may be pedantic, but he is never without a solid foundation, firm as a rock — his opinions are based on chapter and verse.

The doctors of medicine, alas, despise experience, except their own. Past knowledge, the accumulated knowledge of diseases and their cures is ignored, thrown out as antiquated. The quest goes on for something new, something different. One man pronounces a new medical theory; which in a few years is forgotten and buried. Another man discovers, or thinks he does, something different, and before the first exponent is dead, his ideas are superseded by somebody else's. It is a pity that the medical training does not include a course on Logic and Mental Philosophy as well as Medicine.

The principle of the simile in medicine has been discovered and promulgated several times during the centuries. Hippocrates in the 5th century B.C. used the similar remedy, the remedy which produced the same symptoms and cured the similar disease, but his findings were not followed up. Hundreds of years later, Paracelsus again pronounced its importance, again it was lost. Then Hahnemann was inspired and became its first master and worked out the Law of Similars and its corollary: the single, the minimum dose. Naturally he was not believed and his teaching is still ignored by the majority of the medical schools, which is their loss. Although physics and chemistry are proving afresh the truths of Hahnemann's discoveries, one of them being the power of the infinitesimal.

Curability in medicine, in other words prognosis, is the forecasting of what will happen when a certain disease attacks a human being. The prognosis in such a disease as pneumonia some years ago was less than a fifty-fifty chance that the victim would escape with his life. The attending doctor stood by the sick-bed, adopted the benevolent do-nothing attitude of a watcher, leaving everything to nature and the administration of the ministering angel, the good nurse. An excellent way of shelving your ignorance and passing it on to the nurse; but a bit hard on her, blaming her for any failures. Then the vaccines and serums were tried and found wanting; the latest panacea and cure-all of the modern physicians are the different brands, between 70 and 80, I believe, of the sulphonamide series, which have brought down the rate of mortality from over 50 per cent to a round 8 per cent. These figures do not take into consideration the increased feeling of excessive weakness and illness experienced by the patient while these drugs are working in the system. Nor do they take any notice of the prolonged period of convalescence which is necessary after a bout of pneumonia plus sulphonamide medication in those that survive both, nor the liability of a recurrence of the dread disease within a few months; for the immunity to pneumonia seems to be lowered by the sulpha-treatment. And the enlightened opinion of the medical conclave chooses to ignore the serious after effects, the serious lowering of the health of the individual after a siege of sulphonamide treatment, and such complications as various blood diseases, agranulocytosis and the rest. It might be said now of the physician as it used to be said of the surgeon, 'the operation was a success, but the patient died'; changed to this, 'the disease was cured; the patient nevertheless succumbed within a few months, or even days.'

This is destructive criticism — have I nothing constructive to offer? Oh yes! Homoeopathy, despised and rejected as it is, had a death rate for many years of less than 5 per cent of the pneumonia cases admitted to its hospitals, where only the worst cases were found. This death rate is based on the records of many thousands of cases treated in homoeopathic hospitals, not just a few dozens here and there. If numbers count at all, these records should be studied and noted. In private practice the record of pneumonia cases cured when treated according to homoeopathic laws is much higher — the death rate for pneumonia is just 1.5 per cent in several 1,000 cases. The sulphonamide treatment is not in it at all; nor do you find prolonged convalescence necessary in homoeopathic cases, neither are there any complications, nor obscure blood diseases following after a homoeopathic cure.

Pneumonia is only one of the diseases which show a much higher record of cure under homoeopathic treatment. All along the line, the mortality rate is lower, the morbidity rate is less, that is invalidism is reduced by Homoeopathy. And yet, the doors are closed to the spreading, the broadcasting of this knowledge. They will not believe it; they — the orthodox physicians — cannot do it, therefore nobody else can. That is the attitude which is generally taken up.

Slowly, only too slowly, orthodox medicine is drifting to the 'similarity' principle as laid down, enunciated and proved by Hahnemann and his followers. They are coming dangerously — for them and their beliefs — near to the proof that drugs do cause pathological reactions and subjective symptoms which are similar to recognized disease pictures. In America as the *Lancet* reports, a discussion took place at a medical meeting where the similarity between a curious and comparatively rare nervous disease, myasthenia gravis, and the drug Curare was emphasized. Curare is a South American trailing plant, I believe, which the local Indians have for years used to tip their arrows for poisoning their enemies in the inter-tribal fights and in order to drive off and kill unwanted curious foreign visitors.

Some doctors at this discussion went so far as to say that 'Curare produces artificial myasthenia gravis' — which means 'grave fatal weakness of the muscles'. But they are still lost in the jungle of medical contradiction; for then it is stated, that physostigmine is the specific antidote for Curare intoxication and also relieves the symptoms of myasthenia gravis; note the word 'anti'. They still prefer the treatment by opposites.

Now for some more unconscious Homoeopathy: 'the myasthenia patient is abnormally sensitive to Curare, one-tenth of the average dose required to produce general muscle paralysis, induces a profound exacerbation or increase of the usual symptoms in a myasthenia patient.' To the orthodox doctors this was a new discovery, but one which was already known for some considerable time to the homoeopathic physicians who had proved Curare on healthy people and had produced symptoms similar to myasthenia in these individuals. The allopathic conclusion is that it 'would be useful to have another reagent or test added to the diagnostic armamentarium'. Mind you, Curare is to be used for diagnosis only, not for treatment! and a warning is added that the potential dangers of such a powerful drug as *Curare* to a sensitive and enfeebled person, enfeebled by myasthenia, must be remembered (see the *Lancet*, February 27th, 1943).

Now a woman doctor takes up the story and takes it a step further; she bravely ventured to experiment on herself and thus carried out another demand of Hahnemann's to *try out the action of a drug on a healthy human being*, producing subjective symptoms and particularly mental symptoms. A dangerous step as a medical commentator grudgingly admitted; dangerous to the health of the experimenter. This brave woman on reading about a Curare preparation made by the well-known drug firm, Squire, and seeing that an intravenous injection of the drug relaxed the jaw muscles, thought it might conceivably be useful for a laryngeal test, i.e. oral intubation by direct laryngoscopy. She was given, therefore, an intravenous injection of a large dose (5 c.c.) of Curare with dramatic results. She felt the sufferings of a myasthenia patient. Her vision became so blurred that she almost lost it entirely; double vision set in which lasted for two hours except when strong efforts to concentrate were made. Drooping of the eyelids followed, accompanied by extreme prostration, fatigue, a sense of impending death due to transient sensation of constriction in the throat. Any attempt to sit up produced giddiness relieved by shutting the eyes. The mentality remained normal. The next day the symptoms had passed off except for fatigue. The colour of the face was pale and rather grey. The ptosis of the upper eyelids lasted for two hours, and the jaw muscles were relaxed allowing for an easy examination of the vocal cords with a laryngoscope. After this experiment on herself, this doctor used Curare on several patients to obtain jaw relaxation for laryngoscopic examinations. She does not mention whether any of her patients were seized with similar alarming reactions as her own; such as double vision muscular fatigue, prostration and a sense of impending death.

Here again the suggestion is: just to make use of the action of this drug Curare for diagnostic purposes only; that it might feasibly be used as a means of cure has not entered their mental horizon yet.

Here the link which Hahnemann provided that 'like cures like' has not been found, and, indeed, is not being sought for. The chain is incomplete. What is wanted now in order to prove our contention that our law is right, is a clinical test, or many clinical tests, on patients recognized by the medical profession as suffering from myasthenia gravis. Small doses of one of our potencies of *Curare* should be tried, perhaps starting with the 6th centesimal and rising in a series up to the 30th, and should produce spectacular results. I have no doubts of the results. And why should I? The law has proved correct in thousands of cases, and if a case has not been cured, it does not mean that the law is wrong, it means that the right remedy has not been found and the correct drug necessary for a cure is not known yet.

Curare was proved long before this woman doctor was born, by a homoeopathic doctor and the symptoms produced show that it acts largely on nerve endings of the muscles, producing paralysis of the eye muscles, paralysis of the muscles of expression (face); there is immobility of the face with fixed gaze on waking; there is weakness of the leg muscles which give way on walking; heaviness of the arm with increasing difficulty to play the piano; aching and tiredness of the back muscles. Praecordial anguish with palpitation.

Death is due to paralysis of the respiratory muscles. Such is the proving of *Curare* carried out many years ago.

Now in myasthenia gravis all expression is lost, the facial muscles are paralysed, there is no smile, no twitching of the face, it is a wooden block-like face — the patient stares with a frigid frozen look straight ahead into space. The patient complains that the eyes cannot be kept open for any length of time, the lids drop persistently, and the head is thrown back to correct this inconvenience. There is no frowning or wrinkling of the brows as is usual in cases of ptosis from other causes, for the muscle which produces the wrinkling is weak and paralysed. The muscles round the mouth are affected as well and the patient cannot blow or whistle or even smile properly, the corners of the mouth cannot be raised and you get the nasal smile, the furrow of the smile being above the upper lip. Hence you get a smooth, expressionless face with drooping of the lids, and a tendency to throw back the head. Death occurs, due to the weakness of the respiratory muscles and paralysis.

Now compare this disease picture with the picture produced by the action of *Curare*. It is so similar as to be almost identical. The difference in the two medical schools of thought is evident again. The feverish search in the dominant school is for ways and means of finding out what is wrong with the patient, of improving means of diagnosis; excellent as far as it goes; but the true mission of a doctor is forgotten: this the homoeopath supplies. He looks at symptoms, at drug reactions from a different standpoint. We say they should and do show the way towards a cure. The allopath wants to increase his armamentarium in order to make the diagnosis of disease easier, the first duty or mission of a doctor *to heal* is seemingly forgotten.

I have been interested in myasthenia for a long time; for many years ago I had a young woman suffering from this particular trouble. I diligently searched for a remedy; but I did not have many homoeopathic books at my command, and those I had, did not mention a suitable drug. The patient had attended a well-known nerve specialist at a large teaching hospital and I wrote to him for a confirmation of my diagnosis and for any suggestions for treatment. He kindly answered my letter, agreed with my diagnosis, but as for treatment there was not any, he said. The patient might have lived for years; unfortunately she developed a bronchial infection and died in less than twenty-four hours as her weakened respiratory muscles were unable to raise the phleghm.

What is curable in medicine depends on the system of medicine used. Homoeopathic medication correctly applied, not by rota, makes the prognosis of many diseases more hopeful; it helps nature, instead of hindering it.

A few cases taken at random from my case book will serve to show how true the laws of homoeopathy are and justify the efforts now being made to increase its use among all sufferers.

I will just mention such an obstinate complaint as skin trouble. Skin affections are notoriously difficult to cure and even with homoeopathic treatment it may take many months before the curative forces in the body are enabled to cure the external manifestations of the internal disease by stimulation through the similar remedy. Infantile eczema which comes on at or soon after birth is such a disease; it affects the face, ears and scalp; the skin is inflamed, often raw and produces a sticky or watery discharge. Sometimes it is crusty and scabby, always very irritable and the child is miserable, scratching all the time, so that his hands and arms have to be controlled. Orthodox medicine pins its faith on external medication, lotions, pastes, ointments and what nots, which will and may remove the rash. But such a disappearance is not a cure, the cause of the disease is only hidden, remains latent, and breaks out sooner or later in another form, it may be as asthma or renal disease, etc. This fact can never be emphasized enough.

I came across a case of infantile eczema lately. The child was seen on February 1st, 1943; 4½ months old, weight was 13 lb. 3 oz., which was several pounds under weight. She had been attending for at least six weeks at several hospitals for infantile eczema of the face and scalp. It had been thickly plastered with coal tar ointment and was said to be 'cured'. There was still a rash on her face, in front of her ear, and on the scalp; the skin was thickened and looked angry and inflamed; the child was evidently in pain and suffering, for she was screaming all the time and fretful both day and night. It is difficult to get many symptoms from a skin case, but I was told that she was worse during the night and in a warm room, comparatively comfortable out of doors. *Mezereum* 30, one dose, was given, and the mother was asked not to apply any external treatment; ten days later, there was a gain of a pound in weight and the skin was much improved; the rash was hardly noticeable; no medicine ordered. A week later her weight was 14 lb. 9 oz., the crying at night was worse, she scratched more, though the skin was only slightly reddened. (*Mezereum* 30 repeated.)

On March 3rd, a month after her first visit, she had gained 2 lb. all but an ounce (15 lb. 2 oz.). Her face was clear, but she was scratching again: *Mezereum* 30 repeated.

March 15th in contact with whooping cough. *Pertussin* 12 was prescribed as a prophylactic; face clear.

1.4.43; weight 17 lb. 3 oz.; a gain of 4 lb. in two months; did not develop whooping cough; skin cleared up completely; the urine is strong, and scalds her, and her buttocks are inflamed and red. Remembering that her brother had done well on *Medorrhinum* I gave her a dose of *Medorrhinum* 30; this cleared up the buttocks and the urine did not scald any longer. Weight now 17 lb. 8 oz.

April 8th. There is no sign of any skin trouble; at 6½ months old this child is clear of infantile eczema, which normally, in spite of applications of ointments, persists into the second year, and may not disappear in severe cases until the child is 3 or 4 years old. And with the clearing up of the skin the child's health began to improve as well, she put on weight rapidly, looked well and slept well.

Here again homoeopathic treatment, three doses of *Mezereum* 30 and one dose of *Medorrhinum* 30, supplied the missing link, the cure according to the Law of Similarity, and altered the prognosis. Every case of infantile eczema is not curable by *Mezereum*; there are other remedies. In the initial stages with redness and itching *Sulphur* helps frequently, when blisters form in the second stage, *Rhus tox.* is useful; in the suppurating stage, with scabs and crusts formation, *Graphites* is helpful. In the first stage *Psorinum, Pulsatilla, Belladonna, Chamomilla* may be indicated, according to the symptoms present, so try and get the general symptoms; observe carefully and whichever fits the whole child will cure the local affection. For example, *Pulsatilla* would be needed for the fretful whining child, who likes to be carried about and does not get on too well on rich creamy milk, but gains good weight on half cream or skimmed milk. *Chamomilla* must show the strong mental characteristics of *Chamomilla*. *Psorinum* is the offensive child with a strong body odour who feels the cold unduly.

In the vesicular stage, where there is blister formation, *Rhus venenata, Croton tig.* or *Dulcamara* may be necessary; any one of these may answer better than *Rhus tox.* Watch the symptoms carefully, use no local treatment and when the symptoms are clear, then give whatever remedy is indicated on the whole case.

In the crusty, scabby case with moisture, oozing either as a watery or purulent discharge, you may require *Viola tricolor* or *Mezereum* or *Graphites.* Again observe all the symptoms, both local and general, and then the remedy which covers all the symptoms will be the curative one. *Mezereum* will answer well when you get all or most of the *Mezereum* symptoms, and so on with each of the drugs mentioned.

A girl of 12 was seen a few weeks ago with a cellulitis of the flexor tendon of the index finger, duration of trouble two weeks. The finger, at the site of infection, was swollen and stiff, almost black and tender to touch; temperature 99.8 degrees. *Hypericum* dressings were applied externally and *Hepar sulph.* 30 was given internally. Not much improvement was noticed the next day. An incision was then made under local anaesthesia and a cold *Calendula* dressing was applied, when the girl remarked, in a surprised but pleased voice: 'It is cold, not hot.' On asking whether she preferred it cold, she replied, 'Oh yes, much.' On the strength of this gratuitous information, I gave her *Pulsatilla* 30, night and morning, as *Pulsatilla* prefers and is made better by cold external applications. The result was amazing and astounded the nursing staff as well as myself. The pain disappeared at once, the swelling cleared up, the pigmentation of the finger gave way to a normal pink hue and she could move all the joints freely and with ease in twenty-four hours. I saw her five days later, and the finger was practically healed, except for a superficial raw area. All the movements of the finger were normal, no stiffness, no adhesions of the tendon; though the infection was a deep-seated one and the bone was exposed at the time of the operation. Cured in five days after suffering previously for two weeks, and no subsequent stiff finger. The course of the disease would have been, if I had treated it according to surgical rule of thumb: a discharging, slowly healing septic finger for 2 to 3 weeks, followed by a useless stiff finger. This septic finger was cured by homoeopathic medicine in under a week, with complete restoration of all its physiological functions. This is very important to a man or woman in the working classes, for a stiff right index finger is of great hindrance to a woman having to earn her own living by the labour of her hands, and more so to a man.

I remember reading an important monograph by a well--known surgeon some years ago on the treatment of septic fingers and sepsis of the hand, giving minute instructions of how to make the best of a bad job and how to preserve the usefulness of the fingers. This entailed massage, light treatment and galvanic current in order to break down adhesions and meant weeks of out-patient attendance. What a difference under homoeopathic treatment, once you know how to apply the right remedy. No antiseptics were used at all here, the scalpel was placed in methylated spirit prior to use; *Calendula* lotion only was used for dressing the finger before and after the incision, and a few small pills of the indicated remedy, in this instance *Pulsatilla*, were given.

What is curable in medicine was seen some months ago in a middle-aged woman, with a very painful varicose ulcer extending from the ankle upwards for six inches; duration four years. All sorts of treatment had been tried without success. At last the treating practitioner suggested taking out the veins at the knee above the ulcer as a last desperate resort. The woman refused and the doctor prophesied all kinds of dire results. Somebody introduced her to Homoeopathy. In three short months the leg was healed and the deep ulceration was cured, showing but the slightest trace of pigmentation and no deep depression of the scar, which moved freely and easily without any attachment or adhesions to the adjacent bone, the tibia. A most unusual result, usually there is deep staining of the leg, and adhesions to the tibia and deep hollowing where the ulcer has been. And the treatment was very simple. Just *Calendula* lotion, 1 in 10, applied locally; *Calendula* ointment round the ulcer, and the same ointment when the ulcer was healing all over its surface. Internal medication was *Pulsatilla* 6, three times daily for six weeks, then *Pulsatilla* 12 night and morning. No rest in bed was ordered, and the woman had hardly been able to walk outside her own house without the greatest of pain and discomfort for years. Now she can walk for miles, does her own shopping and housework. This happened nearly six months ago and the cure still holds good. Prognosis by ordinary methods was bad in this case: years of ill-health and much suffering were in front of her. Yet this was curable by Homoeopathy, rapidly and painlessly, in a few short weeks. Unfortunately this woman's home-life was extremely unhappy, her husband was cruel and unkind to her and she required treatment for her nerves at intervals for years.

Whatever the name of the disease, it may be myasthenia gravis or some other curious nervous affection, or skin affection, or any disease you like, the missing link, the curative drug, will be found through the study of the action of the drugs on healthy people, and the prognosis of the disease will in many instances be altered and its course will be shortened greatly to the advantage of the sufferer.

CHAPTER TWENTY-NINE

WHAT IS CURATIVE IN MEDICINE

Homoeopathy is considered by the orthodox medical profession as quackery and charlatanism; the most some of them will admit, with a slightly condescending gesture, is that Homoeopathy cannot do any harm, if it does not do much good, as the doses are too minute to have any effect, thus demonstrating their ignorance both of the action of the drugs and the reaction of the people to such remedies.

For example, Dr. Haggard, Professor of Applied Physiology at Yale University – one of the most famous Universities in the United States of America – writes that the secret of the success of Homoeopathy lay not in the effects of the drugs used, 'for these drugs were administered in amounts too infinitesimal to have any effect. Homoeopaths practically gave no medicine at all,' he claims, for though Hahnemann advanced the belief that the smaller the dose the greater the effect, Dr. Haggard considers that he should have said 'the better the results', not 'the greater the effect'. The excessively large doses of potent and often poisonous drugs the medical profession gave at the time of Hahnemann were doing positive harm to their patients, while the homoeopaths achieved their results by just keeping their patients in bed and allowing 'God to do the healing'. In other words, the patients of the allopaths died of the cure and the patients of the homoeopaths died of the disease.

Dr. Haggard used the past tense; according to him the modern methods of 'scientific medicine' are more successful in determining the curative value of drugs, with which optimistic statement some of us might be inclined to quarrel. Many of us think that numbers of patients still die of the cure rather than of the disease. During the Influenza epidemic of 1919 from 20 to 40 per cent of the patients treated by allopathic doctors died, after being treated according to the Modern Scientific Branch of Medical Art. While the homoeopathic physicians lost only 1 per cent of their cases; an outstanding difference of from 19 to 39 per cent in favour of the despised homoeopathic treatment which Dr. Haggard would have us believe had only a brief vogue. Strangely enough Homoeopathy is still going strong and has not been replaced yet by scientific medicine which is based on the specific action of drugs, i.e. a specific drug for each specific disease. The scientific method of proving the specific drug is by controlled mass observation of drug treatment in hospitals. It is not sufficient according to this theory that a patient gets well under a particular treatment, 'he might have got well without it or even in spite of it'. Therefore, the scientific method is to take a certain drug, A, administer the drug to, say, 50 or 100 or more patients, suffering from the same disease, and keep a record of the number who recover, and as a control keep a record of the number of recoveries among the same number of people, suffering from the same disease who are either left to nature or at any rate not given drug A, and then compare results.

If drug A cures a larger number of cases of the particular disease in question, it is a proof that it is the specific drug for that specific disease. Based on this scientific method by mass observation, Mercury was considered to be the specific drug for syphilis for many years, then Salvarsan, discovered by Professor Ehrlich, replaced Mercury, also based on this scientific control method. Lately Salvarsan or 606 has been found wanting and other chemicals for the time being are used in mass experiments, and by the scientific control method large numbers of invalids already weakened by disease are further disharmonized by huge doses of potent drugs. This method of determining the curative value of drugs is completely wrong from the homoeopathic standpoint. Each drug should be tried out on a number of healthy people first; mass observations, yes, but on healthy individuals, and not on sick people, so as to determine the sphere of the action of each drug before trying it out on ill or disabled folk.

The homoeopathic physicians following Hahnemann's lead, have confirmed his contention that there are no specific drugs for specific diseases, but only a specific drug for the particular patient at the precise moment he is being treated, the curative action of the particular drug having been determined first by the effects and reactions it produced on the healthy: this being the simile principle. It is a moot point whether it is more scientific to make mass observations on sick people by means of the control method with a drug whose actions and depths of actions are unknown, or giving a drug to a patient, the action of which has been carefully studied and determined beforehand. With the first method, the so-called modern scientific one, the patient may be extremely sensitive to the particular drug or it may not affect him at all. Nobody knows for certain, until it has been tried out on him. Nobody knows how far and how deep the drug will act, what latent effects it will produce, what secondary effects will follow, what complications will ensue. For example, the sulphonamides have been given by this modern control method, they have reduced the mortality of pneumonia cases, but the list of diseases produced in many people who are sensitive to their action is ever growing. The same with Penicillin. It is being tried in hundreds and thousands of cases. Mass experiments in the army are being done, the scientific mind revels in large figures, so many thousand control cases are at hand ready to be experimented with. It will be a year or more before we shall hear of the failures. It has been ever thus with the scientific method of the curative and specific action of a drug. If I were the patient in question I should refuse to be experimented on, and should prefer the more humane homoeopathic method which heals without any after effects or complications which might not show for months.

What is curative in medicine? Curative in medicine means what is the curative principle in medicine, or what produces the cure? Therefore this implies the therapeutic or treatment side of a physic or drug. Professor Haggard will not admit the value of reporting clinical cases cured under a certain treatment and with a certain drug. I disagree with him entirely; cures based on treatment given according to a definite law should be made known; for 'by their fruits ye shall know them'.

I shall proceed therefore to quote a few cases which were allopathic failures and then cured by medicines given according to the homoeopathic law, that like cures like, and in such doses that the curative or healing action of the drug was brought out.

At the request of the patient a local doctor sent up a case of chronic uncompensated mitral disease of long standing, not because he 'had any doubt of the diagnosis or the treatment' but because his advice of six month's complete rest was not acceptable to the patient. A man about 30, who had not been to school since he was 11 years old, as he spent a great deal of time in bed, due to curvature of the spine after a fall. At 17 he had rheumatic fever and after 15 weeks in bed got up with a bad heart, from which he had never fully recovered. He had done light jobs, but could not hold them for any length of time. Frequently he had to take days off from work as he felt too ill to do any, or he crawled to work, barely able to do a thing. Always very sleepy, he used to collapse in a chair when he got back from his job at night and go to sleep from sheer exhaustion. His symptoms were: still very rheumatic, worse during changes of weather, always worse before rain — recurrent crops of boils, deep scars on back and chest. Septic pimples now showing all over his body, crusts and cracks behind lobe of right ear, which had been discharging off and on for years; is totally deaf on his right side, cannot hear a watch tick holding it close to the ear. Shortness of breath, he was puffing and panting on coming upstairs and took several minutes to recover his breath. Cannot carry any weights at all, chokes when carrying anything; weakness and sagging of abdomen, has to wear a belt for comfort. Heart is dilated, extends outside the nipple line in the 7th interspace; presystolic and systolic murmurs at the apex. Systolic murmur all over the praecordium. Blood pressure 100-50, rather soft pulse, fairly regular, 72. Slight cyanosis of lips and ears; skin greasy and seborrhoeic. Generally worse in damp weather and changes of weather, worse hot weather, worse onions, worse rich food, dreams of falling and wakes up with a start. Vaccinated once in childhood.

What remedy did I choose on these symptoms? First there was the history of rheumatic fever, usually due to streptococcal infection, followed by frequent attacks of boils. On this basis I considered that the streptococcus should be antidoted first and I ordered therefore *Streptococcus* 200th potency, 8 doses, one dose to be taken every tenth day; if improvement should be very striking, the intervals between the doses were to be lengthened. *Thuja* 6, three times daily, was to be taken as well, between the doses of *Streptococcus*, as there were a number of *Thuja* symptoms (worse onions, a greasy skin, dreams of falling, worse sympathy, etc.). *Thuja* 200, one dose to be taken after 3 months' treatment. He was to come back in 6 months, unless there was any change for the worse.

And the result after 6 months' treatment, during which I did not see or hear anything from him? Gain in weight well over a stone; feeling very well in spite of an attack of influenza just before Christmas. Hardly any shortness of breath, even going upstairs; can carry his little girl, aged 4, who is plump and hefty, without any trouble. Skin much clearer, not so greasy, no septic pimples. Deafness of right ear greatly improved, can hear people speak distinctly without having to turn his head or look at them. Can hear a watch with a very soft tick at 2 inches from the ear (has not heard on the right side for years previously). Rheumatism much better, kneecaps slightly affected, weakness and sagging of abdomen greatly improved, sleeping well, dreams not troublesome now. No seborrhoea of ears. The skin which had not been working for years acts freely; a very good thing, as it carried off so much of the impurities.

And he has been working steadily for 3 months, without having a day off, does not feel so exhausted when he gets home, does not go to sleep in the chair now, is not so snappy and irritable – hardly any palpitations. Functional improvement excellent, what about his heart? This was found to be much smaller, the apex beat was in the 6th interspace in the nipple line, pulse strong and even; no presystolic or systolic murmurs, except a slight impurity over the aortic area. B.P. = 115-70. Altogether a most satisfactory result.

Heart disease for 17 years, even since an attack of rheumatic fever. His panel doctor, who had known him for years, told him from his past experience of similar cases that he would never be able to work properly and certainly it would be 6 months before he would be able to do light work even. Instead of which he went back to work after 3 months' rest and kept at it, worked harder than he had ever been able to do all his life without a breakdown. The results astonished me more than I can say. Mitral disease of the heart, which was not well compensated, recovered rapidly after homoeopathic treatment, in spite of having afflicted this man for so many years, when Digitalis and the other heart remedies had not helped him. Homoeopathic treatment was not directed to the heart specially; the remedies were given on the symptoms presented by the individual. The totality of the symptoms showed that *Thuja* was indicated after the septic element was eradicated, for which *Streptococcus* was given for a few weeks. A nosode like this is often a short-cut in homoeopathic treatment and opens the way to the indicated remedy to do its work. The curative principle in this medicine *Thuja*, which improved *this* man out of all knowing, and did so much more than all the so-called scientific drugs of the orthodox school, was based on the Hahnemannian law of similars, which says, 'like cures like'. The symptoms of *Thuja*, the distinguishing particulars, were brought out by healthy individuals who took it in repeated doses and produced such symptoms as the particular type of dream mentioned, the peculiar reaction to changes of weather and to onions, the dislike of sympathy and many other symptoms. *Thuja* was never given to animals in the laboratory in order to produce pathological changes; nor was it first given to sick individuals to see how they would react to it. This is how all the modern drugs are worked out. First in the test tubes on bacteria, secondly on different laboratory animals, and thirdly and lastly on the sick person, already weakened and lowered by his disease.

Thuja has never produced heart disease in an animal and therefore could never be prescribed on physiological grounds. *Thuja* is certainly not a heart remedy in the true sense of the word; but it is curing this man's heart, so that he is able to earn a decent living and enjoys doing it. Because *Thuja* was homoeopathic, that is, similar to the symptoms this man showed; not the physiological symptoms, not the symptoms common to heart disease: shortness of breath, palpitations, inability to carry weights; but the strange, rare and peculiar symptoms, which denoted this particular man: the aggravation after onions, the special dreams of falling into a pit, and so on. This was the curative principle in this medicine for this man and it did and is doing its work well. And so in every new case which presents itself to a homoeopathic physician, he has to start from zero, he has *to know* the patient before him, all his peculiarities, all his oddities, all the hundred and one things which distinguish that particular individual from all the others of the species. Three years later; this man's heart has recovered completely; he has been able to carry on without any break-down, and without having to take any more medicine.

(2) Now another case to illustrate the curative principle in medicine, the reason for selecting a remedy or remedies. This was a man of 63, looking older than his age, short, grey-haired, sallow, dirty yellowish skin, his eyes were tinted with yellow, his tongue coated, breath offensive, pyorrhoea present; veins all over the body thickened and enlarged, temporal arteries tortuous and thickened. His chief complaint for which he came was sudden attacks of 'falling asleep' — narcolepsy is the orthodox name. The first attack came on suddenly the week previous, when he fainted (?) suddenly, as he called it, and remained unconscious for ten minutes and felt sleepy and odd for an hour afterwards. This happened

after a conference on Economics in which he had been very interested. His blood pressure was 190-120, much too high for his age, and this high B.P. was presumably the cause of the prolonged black-out after the mental strain of the conference. He was constipated and in the habit of taking vegetable laxatives, liver pills and salts regularly. Served in the 1914-18 War, had a bad knock on his head, then had Malta fever, but not malaria; hay fever for years, which was 'cured' by nasal cauterization. Three weeks ago had slight bleeding from his nose, again pointing to high blood pressure. So far there is nothing much to prescribe on, from the point of view of the curative principle in medicine. He has tendency to a bunion on the right big toe with a good deal of pain and burning. His left middle finger is beginning to contract and the flexor muscle of the left index finger is stiff and there is a movable nodule (size of a pea) in the soft part of the muscle which interferes with the flexion and extension of the finger. Again all pathological symptoms and there is no basis here for a prescription. Now for a further elucidation with a view to finding the correct remedy. The patient has been vaccinated at least four times, not always success-fully — Pointer No. 1. Suffers from claustrophobia, worse close room, worse both heat and cold, likes sugar, very fond of salt, fear of being locked in, cannot stand the windows shut, partly due to a craving for air, partly due to a fear of being shut in; gets easily annoyed. Keen sense of injustice for other people. Non-smoker, non-drinker.

There are present some *Sulphur* symptoms, some *Nux vomica* symptoms. For years he has taken all sorts of remedies for constipation and to antidote this taking of drugs in the past and for his sedentary habits — he is fond of reading, fond of study, fond of arguing — I prescribed first and foremost, *Nux vomica* 30 three times daily for a week. I took him off all his other drugs and forbade coffee of which he was inordinately fond. Then the various vaccinations had to be antidoted and the different inoculations for typhoid, cholera, etc. He was ordered four weekly powders of *Thuja* 30 to start with, after *Nux vomica* had been acting for a week. Seen six weeks later; great improvement generally, had three slight turns of 'sleepiness' preceded by sensations of giddiness; bowels not open too regularly; skin and eyes not so yellow, but blood pressure 170-120 now. The right bunion is getting smaller and not so troublesome, not so painful, is burning less; is beginning to feel 'on top of the world'. He told me he uses creosote mixture for his throat and catarrh, as he is a singer, which I had not known before, and I asked him to stop this. Ordered *Thuja* 200 (6) a dose every 10th day, to continue *Nux vomica* 30 three times daily for the constipation. It was noted that his breath was greatly improved. Ten weeks later had two slight turns of his 'sleepy attacks' on one day, otherwise greatly improved; eyes clear, not so yellow. I forgot to mention a large cauliflower growth on the lower eyelid which had been annoying him for years — this was another reason for prescribing *Thuja*. This large unsightly wart had become much softer and was distinctly smaller, and 'his feet are grand, does not know he has any feet'. Blood pressure 160-80; prescription *Thuja m* every 10th day (6 doses). To continue *Nux vomica* 30 three times daily. There was some pus in the left tonsil and the temporal vessels are less noticeable, not so thickened and tortuous.

Three months later; one slight turn of sleepiness and faintness after a slight cold 2-3 weeks previously, frontal arteries not standing out any more; eyesight improving, no headaches, no constipation, still catches colds easily, bunion almost gone; fingers of left hand not so stiff; palmar contractions of fingers (Dupuytren's contraction) gone; eyes clear, skin clear, no jaundice of body or of eyes. B.P. slightly higher, 170-120. Prescription *Thuja* 10m (1 dose).

Seen after another 3 months. No bad turns since last visit. The middle finger which used to lock is moving freely, the nodule in the Flexor indicis has disappeared, the contraction of the fingers had been gradually coming on for 2 years and disappeared more rapidly than it came. B.P. 160-100; looks much younger, hair is thicker and not so grey. Jaundice gone, wart on left lower eyelid diminishing in size. Feeling very well. Thickened blood vessels gone. *Thuja* 10m.

This man has had 10 months' treatment for narcolepsy, high blood pressure, bunions, Dupuytren's contraction, and long-standing catarrh. No local treatment was used, no internal remedies were given based on the separate pathological conditions present; but the whole man was treated by remedies. First, by *Nux vomica*, which antidoted previous drugs taken, and secondly by *Thuja* in different potencies, which antidoted the vaccinal poisoning and by removing vaccinosis, Lo! the whole being is cured. *Nux vomica* and *Thuja* were both proved separately in repeated doses on healthy subjects; and the numerous symptoms produced by them gave the indications which were used in this individual suffering from a multitude of pathological lesions, the most serious of which were the high blood pressure and the calcareous infiltration, the thickening of the blood vessels.

(3) A little boy aged 3½ had been treated from January to the end of June, 1943, at one of the Medical Training Schools, for severe attacks of nose bleeding which occurred 2-3 times a week and left him tired and exhausted and reduced his red blood corpuscles. He got gradually worse, so that his parents became more and more alarmed. Then the mother remembered she had been extremely anaemic as a child herself and had been cured about twenty years previously by a woman doctor at a dispensary near by. So she came to the same clinic and was not disappointed in her quest for a cure of her only son's suffering. On enquiry it was found that the boy had been immunized early in January against diphtheria, and the epistaxis (nose bleeding) had started some 2-3 weeks later. Nobody had connected these two facts. He was given *Diphtherinum* 30 on June 29th, 1943, his first attendance and received four weekly doses of *Diphtherinum* 30 until July 26th. His weight was 2 st. 5 lb. when first seen; at the last attendance on August 17th, after 7 weeks, his weight was 2 st. 6½ lb., he had gained 1½ lb. The usual rate of gain in a child of that age is 1 lb in 3 months. He had no recurrence of the nose bleeding since the first dose of the diphtheria antidote; his appetite was excellent; he was

lively and cheerful, slept well, his colour was very good, the anaemia had gone! Homoeopathy had achieved in 7 weeks what allopathy — practised not by an obscure panel doctor in a back street in London, but by one of the most eminent of children's specialists at a large medical training school — had not been able to do in 5 months of regular treatment: cure a little child of nose bleeding and subsequent secondary anaemia!

(4) Now let us compare the results of treatment of coeliac disease — this obscure wasting disease of infancy, caused by an inability to digest fat, and characterized by severe attacks of diarrhoea. I know of 6 cases, 4 recent ones and 2 which occurred several years ago; 4 of them died under orthodox treatment, one is just beginning to show signs of improvement, after the consumption of large quantities of bananas for over 2 months, and the sixth case after having had treatment in a children's hospital for 1 year and 8 months was brought out by the parents in a dying condition. Under homoeopathic treatment this child showed signs of improvement within a week (not 10 weeks' as the banana fed child), and after 3 months' treatment had gained 8½ lb. in weight and was eating a normal diet, including fats. When I saw the child later after three weeks' holiday, there were no signs of coeliac disease, in spite of having had a feverish chill and having been under orthodox treatment for it, our clinic being closed, unfortunately. And the same children's department had not recognized the child as being an old coeliac case of theirs. This could be explained by the child's parents having moved to a different address in the interval!

Is there not a vast difference between the results of the two schools? The homoeopath cures a child rapidly, painlesly, of coeliac disease within a few weeks, without any effort on the parents' part, without being a burden on the ratepayers pockets, without having to call on the R.A.F. to bring over bunches of bananas. And the orthodox school treatment comes limping behind with its vaunted cure of 'bananas being the only thing for this serious disease' and takes months to bring about an uncertain result.

Homoeopathy is not spectacular enough, at least the medicines are not spectacular. They are such minute pilules or granules or colourless, tasteless liquids; and the man in the street cannot believe that there is any power in these tiny things. When he finds that the disease he has been suffering from, maybe for years, disappears and leaves him, after a shorter or longer period, after he has been told by a professor in medicine, let us say, that his disease is incurable and nothing more can be done for him, until death, merciful death, breaks the chain of suffering, he must believe the evidence of his senses, that he is well and he calls it magic.

It is not sorcery or witchcraft, however. It is magic, it is true in the real meaning of the word, which is 'superior wisdom' – the knowledge of the wise man or magus, who knows how to find out what can be cured in medicine and what is the curative action of a medicine and how it is produced. The magic or superior wisdom of the action inherent in each drug and how to make available the powerful vibrations of the energy of a drug, so that it corresponds to and annihilates the strong vibrations of the diseases in the human body, was taught first by Hahnemann, the pioneer scientific chemist and observer of sickness in men. He taught that observation of sickness and the course of an illness at the bedside was necessary for the healing and cure of disease by means of medical remedies. The cause of disease and the cure of disease could only be found by studying man in health and in disease and by observing the effects of a drug on man in health. Thus he could and did find the right, prompt and painless way of restoring the sick man to health.

The Delphic Oracle gave this injunction, 'Man, know thyself', and Pope re-affirms it with these words: 'The proper study of mankind is man', both in health and in sickness, I would add. This supreme wisdom should be taught in all medical schools and be placed in big letters at the gates of hospitals and universities and over the desks of the true healers of the future as a constant reminder of the curative principles in medicine.

SIGNS USED

MOTHER TINCTURE Ø
  < Worse, deteriorated condition
  > Better, improved condition.
ARABIC NUMERALS. 1, 3, 6, 12, 30 following the name of a remedy denotes its potency. Names of remedies are printed in italics.
ROMAN FIGURES such as 1m, 10m or cm. indicate the thousand, ten thousand or one hundred thousand potency of a remedy.

GLOSSARY OF MEDICAL TERMS

ADENITIS	Inflammation of a lymph node.
ALLOPATHIC	Orthodox medical practice using drugs.
ALBUMINURIA	Excretion of serum albumin into the urine, usually suggestive of kidney dysfunction.
ANOREXIA	An absence of appetite.
ANTEFLEXED	Bent forward

B

BLEPHARITIS	Inflammation of the eyelids.
BURSITIS	Inflammation of a bursa which is a small sac containing a viscid fluid which acts as a lubricant to moving parts. Housemaids knee, tennis elbow are examples of this type of trouble.

C

CARDIAC	Relates to the heart.
CERUMEN	Secretion of the glands of the external auditory meatus — commonly described as ear wax.
CLAVICLE	The collar bone.
CORYZA	A running cold or catarrhal inflammation of the nasal passages.
CYANOSED	A bluish discoloration of tissue due to insufficient oxygenation of the blood in certain diseases.

D

DIGITALLY	Examination by use of the finger.
DYSPNOEA	Shortness of breath especially on any exertion.

E

EMPHYSEMATOUS	An abnormal distension of tissue by air in diseased conditions of the lungs.
EPIGASTRIUM	The upper centre of the abdomen under the diaphragm.

F

FIBROID	A non-malignant tumour of the womb.
FLEXOR INDICIS	Tendon of the index finger.
FOETOR	Offensive odour.

H

HAEMOGLOBIN	The iron containing pigment in the red corpuscles of the blood.
HEPATIC	Relating to the liver.
HYPERTROPHY	Enlargement of an organ or tissue.

I

INTRAVENOUS	An injection into a vein.
INTUSSUSCEPTION	When one segment of the intestine enter an adjacent section creating a blockage.
INVAGINATED	Ensheathed.

L

LACHRYMATION	or lacrimal — modern — meaning tears.
LARYNGOSCOPY	inspection of the larynx by a laryngoscope.
LYMPHATICS	The capillary lymph conveying tubes.

M

MACULA	Small patchy skin discolorations.
MARASMUS	A wasting state of being.

O

OEDEMA	An accumulation of serous fluid in the tissues.

P

PATHOLOGY	The study of disease.
PERITONITIS	Inflammation of the peritoneum — the inner abdominal lining.
PHARMACOPOEIA	A book of formulae for use in prescribing drugs, herbs or homoeopathic remedies.
PLACEBO	A non active agent to satisfy a patient during a period of treatment.
POLIOMYELITIS	Inflammation of the grey matter of the spinal cord.
POLYPUS	A tumour arising from a mucous membrane within an organ.
PSORA	Latent predisposition to disease.

R

RALES	Abnormal sounds in the chest.
RHINITIS	Inflammation of the mucous membranes of the nose.

S

S.V.R.	*Spiritus vini rectificatus* — Rectified spirit.
SCAPULA	Shoulder blade.
SECUNDUM ARTEM	according to rule.
SEQUELA	After effects.
SIBILI	Whistling sound in bronchial conditions.
SIMILLIMUM	The most like.
STERNUM	Breast bone.
SUCCUS	Juice.
SYMPHYSIS PUBIS	The cartilaginous joint between the two pubic bones.

T

t.d.s.	Three times daily.
TENESMUS	To strain.
THERAPY	A form or type of healing treatment.
TRITURATE	To grind to a powder.

U

UMBILICUS	The navel.
UNIT DOSE	A single dose of a remedy.

INDEX

X